Diet Myths That Keep Us Fat

Also by Nancy L. Snyderman, M.D.

Medical Myths That Can Kill You:
And the 101 Truths That Will Save,
Extend, and Improve Your Life

Diet Myths That Keep Us Fat

And the 101 Truths That Will Help You Shed the Pounds Permanently

Nancy L. Snyderman, M.D., F.A.C.S.

Chief Medical Editor, NBC News

THREE RIVERS PRESS · NEW YORK

Copyright © 2009 by Nancy L. Snyderman, M.D.

All rights reserved.
Published in the United States by Three Rivers Press, an imprint of the Crown Publishing Group, a division of Random House, Inc., New York.
www.crownpublishing.com

Three Rivers Press and the Tugboat design are registered trademarks of Random House, Inc.

Originally published in hardcover in the United States by Crown Publishers, an imprint of the Crown Publishing Group, a division of Random House, Inc., New York, in 2009.

Library of Congress Cataloging-in-Publication Data

Snyderman, Nancy L.
    Diet myths that keep us fat / Nancy L. Snyderman.—1st ed.
      p. cm.
    Includes bibliographical references and index.
    1. Reducing diets.   2. Weight loss.   3. Common fallacies.   I. Title

    RM222.2.S6355 2009
    613.2'5—dc22

                                                          2008050630

ISBN 978-0-307-40616-3

Printed in the United States of America

Design by Meryl Sussman Levavi

10 9 8 7 6 5 4 3 2 1

First Paperback Edition

To everyone who is still battling that last 5 to 50 pounds

Acknowledgments

We all love being part of a team, and I am very fortunate to be working with some all-stars. I have imaginative, smart, inquisitive, hardworking, and fun women who work together as winners, despite being spread all over the United States, from New York to New Jersey to San Francisco to Dallas.

Amy Rennert, my agent, is one of the best idea people in the publishing business. She has a keen sense of who she is and an inner compass that keeps projects focused and growing bigger and deeper. What began as a friendship but necessitated a business agreement continues to be trumped by the friendship.

Maggie Greenwood-Robinson has continued to research, organize, write, investigate, and challenge medical dogma. She juggles interviews, articles, and my time line better than anyone I have ever known. This manuscript would have never made it on deadline had she not been involved.

Heather Jackson remains my extraordinary editor, the calm voice in the midst of the craziness of ideas and time lines. She raises the standard in every book, every chapter, every paragraph, every word. I am so fortunate to be working with her again. Thanks, too, to the rest of the team at Crown for their expertise and support.

And, of course, no project like this would be possible without the two women who keep me honest and on course at NBC News. Ami Schmitz and Kerri Zimmer are the core of my editorial team at NBC. They are smart and sassy and read medical journals better than any two people I have ever known. They are the true brains behind this reporter.

And, to my patients and viewers who continue to teach me and challenge me and bring me ideas, I am forever grateful.

Contents

Contents

Introduction

Very few of us are ever entirely happy with our weight, and I hate the feeling of putting on a few extra pounds. But I've found some healthy and acceptable ways to get down to a healthy weight—things that really work. If you're like I once was—tired of going on and off diets and up and down in weight—I'm going to help you get and stay naturally fit while eating anything you want, not depriving yourself, and appreciating the wonderful body you have.

How can I make such claims? I am a veteran of the diet wars, a doctor, and a reporter. Between medical school, my internship, and my residency, getting pregnant for the first time in my thirties and the second time in my forties, and doing live television, I've done it all: I've starved myself, and I've pigged out; I've binged, dieted, skipped meals, and lived to tell about it.

I subsisted on vanilla wafers and black coffee while serving my residency in pediatrics. I relied on graham crackers and peanut butter during my surgical training. I've been on liquid diets and protein diets—one week this diet, the next week that diet. I've exercised in sauna suits, and I've dieted on carrot sticks. There are times when I spent so much time poking my head in the fridge that my nose got frostbite. Add whatever you've done to this list, and I would understand. But finally, when *diet* became a four-letter word to me, I said, Enough is enough. I started making friends with food.

So now I have an easy rule. I regard food as fuel. I eat foods I like—even some things that might not be so good for me. As a result, I find it easier to lose weight—I just eat a bit less and exercise a bit more and it falls off. I'm not a member of a health club—it's just not my thing. I prefer walking, hiking, or biking outdoors to keep fit. I watch my weight, but I'm not obsessive about it. And I wouldn't deny myself something I really wanted. Every week, I try to enjoy something from each of my four favorite food groups: the chocolate group, the ice-cream group, the pizza group, and the chips group. But most of the time, I choose healthy foods. Do I have a perfect body? Far from it—but I know I'm healthy.

Making friends with food, with diets, and with your body isn't easy. And a big reason is that most of us have been following certain "rules" for losing weight all our lives. These rules come and go. We are fascinated by them; we follow them. We throw out everything we're doing and embrace the latest rule. If it doesn't work, we blame ourselves for messing up. The truth is that these rules are largely "myths," misinformation that is often considered to be true. Nutrition is a fairly new science and it's pretty boring stuff unless you are a dietitian. But the most important thing we all need to remember is it is always changing. That constant change generates loads of myths, many of which I'll explode in this book—myths like calories don't count, carbs are bad, and you can't keep pounds off.

How do such myths start, and why do they continue? Some myths are holdovers from our mothers and grandmothers, such as "Bread crusts will make your hair curly," or "Gum takes seven years to pass through the digestive system." Others come from fad-diet promoters who use only part of accurate nutrition statements but don't tell you the whole story. Most are interested in making a buck, not in helping you lose weight or keep it off. Other times, the media report news based on incomplete research or the half-truths these diet promoters provide. Tips on how to eat and exercise, stemming from the latest pronouncements by anyone wearing a lab coat or looking good in Lycra, have often been made on very weak data. In all fairness, they may have been the best guess at the moment. But you hear them repeated so many times that you forget they were rough guesses in the first place and come to believe they represent hard facts.

When I began my career as a medical correspondent in the 1980s, I was frequently concerned that one day I would run out of medical subjects, including nutrition, to talk about. Back then, I had no way of foreseeing the bewildering and conflicting flood of diet advice that would continue to pour in week after week. Americans have been bombarded with all kinds of conflicting nutrition news: whether it's about cholesterol and heart-healthy diets or lack of fiber as a cause of cancer, whether it's the latest "miracle" supplement or the dangers of sugar and food coloring, or even whether vegetables are as healthy if they're store bought as they are when purchased at the farmers' market. One day, the supplement vitamin E is magic, an antioxidant hedge against heart disease. Then, just as vitamin companies saturate the market with capsules, research shows that vitamin E takers could be more susceptible to heart attacks than those not taking the supplements.

It can seem as if every food poses a risk for cancer—and that every food contains cancer-fighting agents. Several years ago, health experts promoted a low-fat diet for everyone. Then came the high-protein diet in which promoters said fat is fine, but you need to steer clear of carbohydrates. Eggs used to be bad; now they are good. Butter used to be bad; now we know it's better than margarine.

There is so much misinformation and confusion about what to eat. It gets to a point where there is nothing "safe" left in the refrigerator but the ice maker.

As for the shape we're in, we get fat over the course of years, but we want it off by next Thursday. Hardly a week goes by without some expert somewhere issuing a new report declaring that a certain diet or pill or surgery is the latest magic bullet for weight loss. After being a doctor for more than thirty years, having reported on thousands of diet and nutrition stories, and being a professional dieter myself, I can tell you this: *No magic bullet exists.*

What we need is a new and smart strategy for successful weight loss. Statistics show that forty-five million Americans are dieting at any moment in time, and we're spending more than $30 billion a year on weight loss. Yet obesity is rarely treated successfully. We have a serious problem: We are the only animals on the planet that will eat ourselves into an early grave. Two centuries ago, people died of starvation. That trend is changing. Ours will be the first generation to die from food excess. It's insane!

Since the early 1980s, Americans increasingly have grown larger. We are ten pounds heavier, on average, than we were fifteen years ago and eat 15 percent more calories today than in 1984. Adult obesity has doubled since 1980, increasing in every region of the country, in both males and females and across all age, race, and socioeconomic groups. As we grow bigger, so have our risk factors for heart disease, stroke, high blood pressure, type 2 diabetes, gallbladder disease, elevated cholesterol levels, kidney failure, and certain cancers. We're at a tipping point in this country, where obesity has started to cost us our longevity. Proper weight is not just a matter of looking good; it is about health. Being healthy is knowing you can count on your body. Being healthy is about enjoying a well-rounded life: pursuing physical activities you love, enjoying a balanced diet that makes room for all foods in moderation, and tuning in to your emotional and spiritual health.

One answer to our national paunch is to stop obsessing about what we eat and start sorting out the sound advice from the babble. In spite of all the conflicting information, the tried-and-true still holds: Load up on real foods like fruits, vegetables, and whole grains; practice portion control; and exercise regularly. It couldn't be simpler. And because it's so simple, people find it really boring. But these actions are the only safe and stable ways to lose weight.

Try not to react to every new nutritional study that comes down the pike, either, since much of this information will be replaced by a new panacea next month. And start savoring your food, whether it's a steaming bowl of oatmeal or a piece of double-fudge cake you share with your friends at a great restaurant. Food is good for you, and it's good for your soul. Enjoy it!

I feel that beyond being a myth buster, this book should also act as a pal. I can help you most effectively if I give you enough truthful information to guide you out of the confusing diet maze. Then you can say, "Enough is enough. Tomorrow I'm starting on a new course that is best for me." So treat this book as a resource, a constant companion, and a lifetime guide for taking weight off and keeping it off. Many of us have been fed (excuse the pun) bad information about diet, nutrition, and weight loss. Bad information means bad choices, and bad choices mean bad results—or no results. You can't get in shape and stay healthy unless you know the truth.

This book will bring you face-to-face with the truth about dieting and weight loss, and armed with that truth, you'll learn how to:

- **Check out information before you act on it.** For example, if you were told that eating fifteen grapefruits each day would help you burn fat, would you go to the nearest supermarket and stock up? Or would you check it out first?

- **Make informed decisions using sound, straightforward information.** Question whether a popular diet will really work for you.
- **Learn to make a friend of food and exercise.** This will allow you to safely sprinkle the not-so-healthy stuff through your diet and not feel deprived.
- **Understand that being overweight isn't always the result of overeating and underexercising.** There's a lot more to fatness than lack of willpower. For many of you, being overweight is not your fault. Yet there are still many factors that are within your power to change.
  - How you eat can lower your risk of heart disease, stroke, and certain cancers.
  - Discover little-known yet powerful facts and motivating ideas that can keep you trim and energetic.
  - Make important permanent changes—the kind you can live with for the rest of your life—in your eating habits.
  - Escape the forbidden-food mentality, allow yourself some leeway, and learn to enjoy food again with my Treat Yourself Diet—and lose weight in the process.

Whether your weight-loss goal is 5 pounds, 50 pounds, or more, you can achieve it in some of the most enjoyable ways possible—by eating the foods you love in satisfying moderation. It's not about becoming super-model thin or adhering to someone else's ideal, either—it's about being healthy and feeling great. And it's never too late to begin the journey. I am living proof that decades-old diet patterns can, with intervention and commitment, be changed. I am at peace with food. And I want you to be at peace, too.

Myth #1

Your Weight Is Your Fault

The first time I set out to lose 20 pounds, I ate only protein. The second time, I crunched down on raw carrots and swilled diet sodas. Every trick I tried worked for a while, until it didn't. For the longest time, I chalked my failures up to lack of willpower.

I can say with certainty that I've learned a lot since those days, and what I've learned is that weight control is not all about willpower, and it's more than just what you put in your mouth (or don't). Obesity and being over-weight are problems of many causes. There are powerful drives and forces in our lives—social, environmental, and biological—that make it extremely difficult for some people to lose weight. The very behaviors we're trying to adopt—like eating healthfully and exercising regularly—are being actively discouraged by society.

Enlightenment on why we're overweight hit me

square in the face in 2008 when I visited China during the Olympics. I was there to cover the country's health issues for NBC News. My assignments included the obvious, from the treatment of athletic injuries to possible doping scandals, but I was also interested in looking at the Chinese way of life. What did the Chinese eat? Where did they go for health care? How far had high-tech Western medicine encroached on centuries-old Chinese medicine?

I had always thought the Chinese people were slim, petite, and fit, so I was unprepared for what I saw there: a significant number of overweight and obese people, young and old. As I soon learned, China is now the second-fattest country in the world, in second place only to the United States. Curious, I visited a so-called fat-reduction hospital two hours outside Beijing that has an interesting inpatient treatment program for teenagers who are battling fat.

There I interviewed a thirteen-year-old boy, Yi, who was the same age as my son, Charlie. Yi, a lively boy with close-cropped black hair and a toothy grin, was a good 25 pounds overweight. Like growing numbers of Chinese youth, Yi was trying to lose it. "I am spoiled by my parents and my grandparents," admitted Yi, the only child of his family's clan. "They give me sweets, and take me to fast-food places." The obesity issue reflects the new affluence in China and the chance to eat fast food—and an unintended consequence of the one-child policy, where grandparents unconsciously reward behavior with food.

Yi was lying on his back with acupuncture needles poking the area around his belly button. "It hurts a little bit," Yi said, as the acupuncturist twirled the needles in his flesh. The ancient Chinese therapy supposedly works by targeting specific "points" on the body that correspond with your emotions, stress levels, energy (or qi), and physical body.

Yi was losing weight with techniques as old as this ancient land, not only acupuncture but also treatments such as herbal remedies and massage. Doctors had taken him off fast food and put him on the traditional Chinese diet of porridge, rice, vegetables, and a little bit of chicken-wing meat. On an average morning, Yi and other obese teens would undergo their half-hour acupuncture treatment and then engage in light exercise, including badminton or walking. Unfortunately, the hospital weight-loss program was a little weak on the educational side; kids were sent home with only a pamphlet on nutrition and no real program in place for follow-up or maintenance.

"What is the one thing you miss most about being at home?" I asked the youngster.

"I miss fried beef," he said.

I thought to myself, "If this kid misses fried beef, he's probably going to start eating it again, plus other fattening things he loves. The chances of this boy keeping his weight off are not good."

Approximately sixty million Chinese, equal to the population of France, are overweight and obese. In a nation that has for centuries consumed most of its calories from rice and vegetables and is fabled for eating almost every part of a chicken or pig, how could China now be facing an obesity epidemic not unlike our own?

There are three big reasons, and the first one is the

availability of fast food. Kentucky Fried Chicken is the number one fast-food franchise in China, with McDonald's running a close second. As their society has become more affluent, the Chinese have more disposable income, which they dispose of at fast-food restaurants.

Second, because of China's one-child policy, many parents spoil their kids by treating them to fast food and sweets. Today, 5 to 10 percent of the younger generation is regarded as overweight, and the figures are expected to double within a decade.

Third, the country that was recently known as the land of bicycles is quickly becoming the land of the couch potatoes. Instead of bicycling to work, they are driving cars or riding on subways. Millions of urban dwellers are living a sedentary lifestyle, dominated by computers, television, the Internet, video games, and DVDs. Also, because of the pressure from competition to enter good higher schools, teachers sacrifice students' exercise time for class work.

The bottom line is that social, cultural, and environmental forces have all conspired to turn China into a nation of overweight citizens. And of course, that's exactly what has happened in America. Clearly, it's not entirely our fault that we're hungry and heavy. There's a lot more to the story than meets the fork.

ANATOMY OF A MYTH

The need to lose weight has become a part of everyday life, but that hasn't made it an easy goal to achieve. We work at it, struggle with it, battle it, and usually end up extremely frustrated by the whole process. That being said, it is very important to know that you *can* succeed, as long as you understand what you're up against.

On a very simple level, your weight depends on the number of calories you consume, how many of those calories you store, and how many you burn (see Myth #3). But each of these factors is influenced by so much more. Maybe your mom's family has always been heavy. Grandma can't bear to waste food because the world's poor are starving, and your brother Mike wasn't hungry until he saw that TV ad for fried chicken, gravy, and mashed potatoes. Your sister Jane hates to turn down a bargain, and that supersized meal was a super deal. Your uncle Henry only eats things out of packages. And who brought those doughnuts to the office, anyway?

We assume that people are overweight because of personal failings, that they're lazy, weak, and gluttonous, and that they don't have the willpower to eat right or exercise. But there's a growing awareness that heredity, environment, and even factors like increased stress and lack of adequate sleep, can wreak havoc on the body's metabolism, contributing to weight gain. Obesity is now classified by the National Heart, Lung, and Blood Institute as a complex, chronic disease involving many environmental, social, behavioral, metabolic, and genetic factors.

DO YOUR GENES FIT?

Heredity determines, at least partially, how many fat cells your body has and how large these fat cells are. Your genes can affect your physiology (such as how fast you burn calories) as well as your behavior (the types of foods you choose to eat, for instance). They may also contribute to appetite, satiety (the sense of fullness), metabolism, food cravings, and your body-fat distribution.

Several studies have shown that identical twins, separated at birth, have similar body types, including obesity, when reunited years later. It makes sense that genes that determine everything else about us also play a role in obesity.

The strength of the genetic influence on weight problems varies quite a bit from person to person. Research suggests that for some people, genes account for just 25 percent of the predisposition to be overweight, while for others the genetic influence is as high as 70 to 80 percent. Having a rough idea of how large a role genes play in your weight may be helpful in terms of managing your weight. Take my quiz on the next page to get a glimpse at how much your weight depends on your genes—and what you can do about it.

And you can do a lot about it. Your DNA is not your weight-control destiny. Several years ago, I interviewed obesity expert Dr. James O. Hill, one of the researchers who established the National Weight Control Registry, a database of more than five thousand successful dieters who have maintained their weight loss of 30 pounds or more for at least six years. "Over 60 percent of the people in the National Weight Control Registry report that they were overweight as children," he told me. "So it doesn't mean that long-term success in weight management is impossible." Another myth busted: If you're

Quiz: How Much of Your Weight Depends on Your Genes?

Read through each statement below, and answer yes or no to each.

Group A Statements

1. I have been overweight for much of my life.
   ❏ Yes   ❏ No

2. One or both of my parents, or several other blood relatives, are significantly overweight.
   ❏ Yes   ❏ No

3. I can't lose weight even when I faithfully stick to a reducing diet and increase my activity and do this for several months.
   ❏ Yes   ❏ No

Group B Statements

4. I am strongly tempted by the availability of food.
   ❏ Yes   ❏ No

5. I'm moderately overweight, but I can lose weight when I diet and exercise.
   ❏ Yes   ❏ No

6. I tend to gain weight easily if I don't follow a healthy diet.
   ❏ Yes   ❏ No

Group C Statements

7. I've never really been overweight.
   ❏ Yes   ❏ No

8. I can eat almost anything I want and not gain weight.
   ❏ Yes   ❏ No

9. I don't exercise much, and my weight stays normal.
   ❏ Yes   ❏ No

Scoring

- If you answered yes to two or more statements in Group A, genes are probably a significant contributor to your weight issues. For people with a very strong genetic predisposition, sheer willpower can be tough in counteracting the tendency to be overweight. But you can achieve and maintain weight loss under a doctor's guidance (see Myth #6).

- If you answered yes to two or more statements in Group B, genes are probably a lower contributor for you. While you have some genetic predisposition to be heavy, it's not so great that you can't overcome it with some effort devoted to diet and exercise.
- If you answered yes to two or more statements in Group C, your genetic predisposition to obesity is low. You have a good chance of losing weight by eating fewer calories and getting more vigorous exercise. It may also be easier for you to keep it off.

heavy as a child, you'll be obese as an adult. Simply not true!

In the United States, we've been getting fatter since the seventies. The trend is universal and cuts across all demographic groups. So we can't blame such a rapid rise on genes alone. Let's look at another factor—hormones—as a contributor to the epidemic.

TRUTH

Moderately overweight kids shouldn't be put on restrictive diets.

If you have kids who are 10 to 15 pounds overweight, the current thinking is that they should not be put on restrictive diets. Instead, it's better to help them make basic improvements in their diets, ramp up their activity, and give up some TV and computer time. Perk up your kids' diet by adding more fruits, vegetables, and whole grains while cutting back on the junk foods. That way, you'll automatically slow the rate of their weight gain while they continue to grow in height. Children go through dynamic phases of growth, and a low-calorie diet is not what they need. They need nutrients and activity.

IS IT MY HORMONES?

Hormones are complex chemicals produced and secreted by glands that regulate and control the activity of other organs in the body. A hormone is released by a specific gland, travels through the bloodstream, is absorbed by the target organ, and sets off the desired chain reaction. Hormones help control when and how often you feel hungry, how much you eat, even how quickly food is burned as energy. There are many hormones involved in weight regulation, but the two key hormones are leptin and ghrelin.

Leptin

Secreted into the bloodstream by fat cells found in the stomach, leptin is a hormone that tells you when you've eaten enough. Basically, it signals the brain to release hormones that suppress hunger. If you have low levels of leptin, as many people who are obese do, you tend to feel hungry much of the time.

You don't have to be at the mercy of leptin fluctuations, however. To regulate normal production, just make sure you log enough z's. Your body produces the hormone while you sleep. Plus, ample evidence shows that eating fatty fish like salmon, mackerel, or sardines increases leptin levels and may help you keep your weight down. Ease off saturated fats in your diet, too. They cause your body to release less leptin. Saturated fats are the artery cloggers found in foods that come from four-legged sources: high-fat red meats, butter, full-fat cheeses, and other whole-milk products. Finally, moderate your alcohol intake. More than one drink a day for women and two drinks daily for men can make leptin levels drop.

Ghrelin

Ghrelin is secreted into the bloodstream by stomach glands. It signals the brain to secrete hunger-stimulating hormones, and you start feeling hungry. When you diet, ghrelin levels rise and leptin levels fall. Your appetite increases, making it harder to lose weight.

Fortunately though, it's easy as pie to tame ghrelin and prevent it from triggering a feeding frenzy. From what we know now, it seems that all you have to do to keep ghrelin down is to stay moderately full and avoid getting really hungry. How do you do that? One of the best ways to regulate your appetite and still lose weight is to eat three healthy meals a day, with nourishing snacks in between. Multiple meals of beneficial foods are linked to lower body fat, better-regulated hunger hormones, and the steady release of blood sugar throughout the day to help calm cravings.

My message here is, yes, hormones regulate weight, but that doesn't mean you don't have a say in the matter. You do. Take the upper hand by choosing the right foods, not skipping meals, and eating frequently throughout the day.

OUR FOOD-FOCUSED WORLD

While genetic factors and hormones are those forces inside you that can mess with your weight, environmental factors are the outside forces that contribute to the problem. They encompass anything in our environment that makes us more likely to eat too much or exercise too little.

Practically everywhere we go—shopping centers, gas stations, sports stadiums, movie theaters—food is readily available. You can buy snacks or meals at roadside rest stops, twenty-four-hour convenience stores, and even gyms and health clubs. We are surrounded by processed foods that are higher in fat and sugar at the expense of grains and fiber. Not surprisingly, we're also eating more high-calorie foods (especially salty snacks, soft drinks, and pizza), which are much more accessible than lower-calorie choices like salads and whole fruits.

Back in the 1950s and early 1960s when I was growing up in Fort Wayne, Indiana, fast-food restaurants offered one portion size. Now there are multiple portion

TRUTH

Weight gain after a splurge isn't all fat.

The day after your splurge, you may weigh two to four more pounds, but this increase is primarily water weight gain. Extra carbohydrates are stored primarily as glycogen, and for each ounce of glycogen you'll store about three ounces of water. This water weight comes and goes within a day or two. Excess calories from fat are stored as body fat. But keep in mind that a single pound of fat is the equivalent of 3,500 excess calories. That's a lot of food (about seven Big Macs or eighty chocolate-chip cookies) above your normal intake—not just a mere slice of cheesecake. All you have to do is get back on track with your normal eating plan, and those pounds you see on the scale will drop right off.

sizes, and those sizes verge on the gargantuan. A typical serving of french fries from McDonald's contains three times more calories than when the franchise began. A single supersized meal can contain 1,500 to 2,000 calories—all the calories that many people need for an entire day. And research shows that people will often eat what's in front of them, even if they're already full.

Americans are eating more calories on average than they did in the 1970s, says the Centers for Disease Control and Prevention. Between 1971 and 2000, the average man added 168 calories to his daily fare, while the average woman added 335 calories a day. (Do the math: If you're "average," that translates into a gain of nearly 20 to 50 pounds a year!) Incidentally, I don't know why women added more calories than men, but I suspect it may have to do with emotional eating. Women tend to eat emotionally; men do not.

Dietary fat isn't necessarily the problem, either. Research shows that the fat content of our diet has actually gone down since the early 1980s. But many low-fat foods are very high in calories because they contain large amounts of sugar to improve their taste and palatability. In fact, many low-fat foods are actually higher in calories than the foods they're replacing.

As for physical activity, it's almost impossible to find a staircase to use in place of an elevator; and we drive everywhere instead of walking because there aren't any sidewalks or it's too far to walk. We sit while we work and use labor-saving devices like moving walkways, automatic doors, remote controls, drive-through windows, and other "conveniences." Computers make it possible to communicate, shop, play games, and socialize without lifting more than your fingers. Because we work long hours, we have trouble finding the time to go to the gym, play a sport, or exercise in other ways.

And our kids? We're so afraid to let them outside unsupervised that they get little outdoor time. Instead, they stay inside playing video games and watching TV. As for activity at school, gym classes have been dropped at many schools.

Experts think that taken together, environmental factors are the driving force for the dramatic increase in obesity. Yet these factors are totally within our power to change. Some suggestions:

- **Reclaim what technology has stolen from you.** Move your wastebasket to the other side of your office, lose the remote control, put your recycling bin as far away from your kitchen as possible. Avoid buying appliances and outdoor yard equipment that use electricity or gas when a manual option is available and reasonable.
- **Clear out high-calorie, tempting binge foods from your pantry or refrigerator.** Everything that threatens to wreck your resolve, including ice cream, leftover pie, and pizza, must go. If it's there, you'll be tempted to eat it—so toss it or hide it in a container. If you don't see it, it's much easier to avoid.
- **Don't go grocery shopping when you're hungry, and avoid the snack-food aisles.** Buy only healthy foods and stick to a shopping list. If

TRUTH

You can lose more weight in cold weather.

Some people swear they gain more weight in the wintertime. Frankly, I think it's because we're not quite as active in winter. But the reality is, your metabolism revs up to keep your body warm in cold temperatures. This may mean marginally more calorie expenditure each day.

you must buy fattening foods for the nondieters in your family, purchase versions you don't like. If you covet chocolate-chip cookies, buy another type of cookie for your family instead.

- **Avoid situations that trigger overeating.** Choose a route to and from work that doesn't involve passing your favorite fast-food restaurant, ice-cream parlor, bakery, or any other place that has caused trouble in the past. Keeping your finger off the trigger can go a long way toward helping you lose weight.

OBESITY SPREADS

Even our friends can make us fat! Research from Harvard Medical School says that obesity can be socially contagious; in other words, having fat friends or family around can make you fat. This doesn't mean obesity is contagious in the sense of "catching it" the way you catch a cold or flu. But a friend's weight may indeed influence your eating and your thinking.

According to this landmark study, if your close friend becomes obese, your chances of becoming obese increase 57 percent; if your siblings are fat, the increase is 40 percent; and if your spouse is hefty, the increase is 37 percent. One explanation is that friends affect each others' perception of fatness. When a buddy becomes obese, being fat may not look so bad. We're also influenced by other people's eating habits; when everyone around us is eating, we join right in. On a better note, weight loss is also contagious: if you hang around with thin people, you're more apt to be thin.

To avoid getting fat by association, try the following.

- **Include your family and friends in your weight-loss efforts.** Cook healthy meals for your whole family. Start a walking group in your neighborhood or form a healthy-recipe dinner club. Find a gym buddy so you can motivate each other to get fit—it's likely your friends could use the boost, too, since less than 50 percent of Americans do nothing to keep fit.
- **Join a group-centered weight-loss program, like Weight Watchers, rather than go on a diet by yourself.** These groups provide a built-in social network of people working toward a common goal. Research has shown that it's easier to quit smoking, stop drinking, and lose weight in programs that provide peer support.
- **If none of your friends is interested in exercise or eating well, seek out some who are.** Alternatively, consider hooking up with an Internet

support group designed for people interested in health and fitness. But *don't* ditch your heavier friends. That's taking things too far for any diet. Also, there is plenty of research that suggests having more friends makes you healthier.

STRESS CAN MAKE YOUR WAISTLINE BULGE

When the going gets tough, I have, like countless other people across America, been known to get eating. A rapidly approaching deadline at work? Toss me that bag of chips. Feeling overwhelmed with my home to-do list? A few of those chocolate-chip cookies will do the trick.

Feelings of stress, anxiety, anger, sadness, loneliness, or even joy send many of us straight to food. But why are so many people driven to use food as an emotional salve? Part of it may be physical: We know that certain things like carbohydrates boost levels of serotonin, a feel-good brain chemical. Also, on a very basic level, most of us associate food with comfort, ever since Mom soothed us with warm milk when we were babies or a bowl of chicken soup when we were sick. The other part is habitual: Handfuls of M&M's comforted us once before, so they'll help again now.

In some cases, your stress may even make your kids heavier. A new study published in the journal *Pediatrics* looked at the relationships in low-income families regarding kids' weight, the availability of ample food in their homes, and their mothers' stress. Researchers found that kids ages three to ten in "food-secure" homes whose mothers reported feeling stressed were more likely to be overweight than kids in "food-insecure" homes with similarly stressed-out mothers. "Food security" is a term used by the Department of Agriculture to describe the degree to which a household has access to enough food to sustain healthy, active lifestyles for everyone in the family. The researchers speculated that in stressful environments, kids reach for comfort food more often.

There's more: Stress causes weight gain in the tummy by triggering the brain to release the hormone cortisol to ready the body for "fight or flight." High levels of cortisol increase the appetite, typically for carbs and fats. Visceral, or deep-layer, fat in the abdomen has more receptors for cortisol than fat elsewhere in the body, causing your body to lay down more flab, especially around the middle.

Fortunately, cortisol drops when you boost endorphin levels with a massage, meditation, or exercise. Exercise is one of the best stress relievers around. When things get overwhelming and tense for me, nothing is better than getting my heart rate up and sweating. I will try to get out of the house and take a very brisk walk or a run. I think fresh air and a change in locale help clear the brain. I've come up with some of my best solutions to problems when I've used this escape strategy.

For weight control and peace of mind, you need to practice all those stress busters you've heard about, such as deep breathing and meditation. Another great stress buster is learning to say no and mean it, in much the same way you say no to fattening food. People today are so busy fulfilling multiple responsibilities, whether it's as a parent, spouse, employee, or friend, they forget about themselves. If you want to handle your stress, heck, if you want to live a rich and full life, you must start putting your needs on the front burner. There's a reason the airline attendant instructs you to put on your oxygen mask before you put on your child's. If you don't look after yourself, you won't be of much use to others.

One of my favorite professors once told me that time is our most valuable commodity, and others will waste it for us if we let them. So I no longer let them. Now I set priorities realistically and say no when I really mean it.

If you're an emotional eater, here are some other strategies to help you.

- **Keep a food journal.** Writing down what you eat, as well as when you eat, can clue you in to patterns that cause mindless eating. You'll discover what's precipitating your eating—whether it's disappointments, daily activities that cause more stress, or simply fatigue.
- **Find substitute activities.** When you know what triggers emotional eating, you can replace eating with something else. Have handy a list of what you can do besides eat to feel better: take a walk, read a good book, call your best friend, enjoy a bubble bath, work on a hobby, or exercise. Use this strategy and you'll definitely feel (and see) a difference.
- **Schedule your eating.** Having a set meal and snack schedule can help you avoid impulse eating. Try to eat three regular meals with scheduled nutritious snacks if you find yourself becoming hungry between meals. If you're not hungry but

TRUTH

Hypnosis is useful for stress eating.

While hypnosis in itself cannot make you lose weight, some people are using hypnotherapy to help them become more relaxed and less stressed so that they won't binge or eat emotionally. This in turn helps them make the changes necessary to lose weight and keep it off

an urge to nibble hits you, wait fifteen minutes or so; it may help distract you until the impulse passes.

- **Seek professional help if your stress continues or you cannot overcome emotional eating on your own**.

SLEEP YOURSELF SLIMMER

In 2004 I hosted a special on ABC called *Sleep: How to Get the Rest of Your Life*. Doctors from the Stanford Sleep Disorders Clinic put me through a grueling three-day sleep-deprivation regimen, to demonstrate how much one's memory, reaction time, and abilities can be impacted by lack of sleep. At the end of my seventy-two-hour sleep drought, I drove around a special course at the Infineon Raceway near Napa to demonstrate the resulting impairment. I was astonished. I was deluded enough to think that I was more in control than I really was, but I drove like someone who was drunk. Even more to my surprise, I also gained three pounds.

Weight gain is one of the most disturbing consequences

of lack of sleep. Insufficient sleep tends to disrupt hormones (including leptin) that control hunger and appetite. The optimal amount of sleep for weight control is between seven to eight hours a night. If you sleep fewer than six hours most nights of the week, you can put on up to 11 pounds over six years, say various studies. That may not sound like a big deal, but it can add to the creep of obesity caused by other factors such as stress or lack of activity.

I know there is no substitute for a good night's sleep. In the modern world, we work hard to live life to the fullest, cramming as much as we can into our waking hours, assuming we'll catch up on sleep later. But the reality is, you can't catch up on sleep. Once it's gone, it's gone. Trying to make up for it on the weekend is a poor strategy that usually backfires in a bout of insomnia on Sunday night. Sleep is a daily need and should be treated as such. If you have regular difficulty sleeping, sit down with your doctor and try to figure out what's wrong. Our sleep cycles can be disturbed for a million reasons. Are you under stress? Depressed? Has your life shifted to late dinners out with too much wine and not enough exercise? Have you been traveling across time zones? These can all cause sleep problems.

A lot of people think sleeping pills are the answer—and they can help in the short term—but there are lifestyle changes you can make, too, and that you should try first. Staying away from stimulants like sugar, caffeine, nicotine, as well as avoiding alcohol before bedtime, can make a difference. Avoid stimulation like computer work or exercise for at least three hours before going to bed. But if you exercise earlier in the day, it can improve your sleep at night. Establish a relaxing bedtime routine. For me, it's reading a medical journal in bed. And do go to bed at the same time each night. Clean up your sleep habits. You'll look better and feel better.

EXTRA, EXTRA

Family meals prevent eating disorders.

Anorexia, bulimia, and binge eating are eating disorders that have increased steadily over the decades, mostly in young women—though no one is really immune. I had a college roommate, Lisa, who was an accomplished ice skater. One year, after Christmas break, her coach made a comment about a rival skater, noting that she was tall and thin and graceful. That was enough for Lisa to interpret the comment as an insult and she stopped eating. By the time we graduated, she was down to 67 pounds and hospitalized. Years after college I saw her, and thankfully she had worked through her eating disorder and was at a normal weight.

I was happy to see a recent study in the *Archives of Pediatrics and Adolescent Medicine* that shed light on one way to prevent eating disorders: family meals. The study found that teenage girls who frequently eat meals with their families are less apt to use laxatives, diet pills, and purging to control their weight. Interestingly, family meals didn't make a difference when it came to boys, though girls were three times as likely to use dangerous dieting behaviors in the first place. The researchers don't know why but speculate that girls might need the family bonding time more than boys do. This piece of research underlines the importance of making time for the family meal, where everyone sits down and eats together. Let's bring this tradition back from the verge of extinction.

DIETING WITH YOUR DOCTOR

There are so many factors to blame for obesity and being overweight that I'm a big believer in seeing your physician about weight problems. Doctors are much more savvy about weight control than they used to be. Of course, not everyone needs to see a doctor to lose weight, but some people might want to consider this option for two reasons. The first is to get medical guidance. If you haven't been able to lose weight on your own by dieting and exercising, your doctor may be able to diagnose why and help by making specific recommendations. The second is to be evaluated for health complications that might be linked to your excess weight.

Chances are, your primary care physician can perform this evaluation. Depending on what your doctor finds, he or she may refer you to a dietitian to assess your eating habits, or to a therapist to address any psychological issues that may be promoting weight problems. If you're overweight and have weight-related complications, your doctor may refer you to a medical group that specializes in weight loss or to a hospital-based weight-loss center.

Your doctor will ask you about your lifestyle: how much you eat and drink and whether you're a charter member of the couch-potato club. I realize it's embarrassing to admit to some bad habits, but we doctors have heard it and seen it all before. Hold nothing back. Your doctor has the right to know the truth about your habits. Admit to the fatty food, the alcohol, and cigarettes. Tell

TRUTH

Having regular saunas will not help you lose weight.

People still believe this old wives' tale that we lose weight by having saunas. Yes, we weigh less after a sauna, but this is because we sweat. The lost fluid is gradually replaced through the day when we drink water or other beverages.

him about the herbal medications and over-the-counter products you are taking. They can affect treatment.

Your doctor will also be interested in knowing what you've tried on your own to lose weight. What diets have you followed? Did you lose weight on any of these plans? How long did you keep off the weight, and how much did you regain? This information can help your doctor determine strategies that might be more successful, so be honest.

In addition to your personal history, your doctor will query you about your family medical history. For example, do you have a family history of disorders that can be caused by obesity, such as type 2 diabetes or high blood pressure? If so, you might be at high risk for these problems.

As part of your medical history, give your doctor the names of all the medications you've been taking. Several drugs can cause weight gain, increase appetite, or interfere with your weight-loss efforts. If your weight gain came on soon after you began taking one of these drugs,

Drugs That Cause Weight Gain

Lots of prescription drugs can cause weight gain by increasing your appetite or slowing your metabolism. If you suspect that a drug you're taking might be affecting your weight, notify your doctor. He or she should be able to adjust your dosage or switch you to a drug that doesn't have this frustrating side effect. Here's a partial list of drugs known to have the side effect of weight gain.

Corticosteroids

Estrogen and progesterone

Anticonvulsants, such as valproic acid

Certain anticancer medications

Antidepressants, including lithium; tricyclic antidepressants, such as imipramine (Tofranil) or desipramine (Norpramin, Pertofrane); monoamine oxidase inhibitors; and selective serotonin reuptake inhibitors, such as paroxetine (Paxil), citalopram (Celexa), escitalopram (Lexapro), sertraline (Zoloft), fluvoxamine (Luvox), and fluoxetine (Prozac).

Insulin

Glyburide

it may be the cause of your problem. Depending on your condition, you may not be able to stop taking the drug, but you might be able to substitute it and lose the extra weight.

A few illnesses can make you gain weight, too. These include hypothyroidism (an underactive thyroid); polycystic ovarian syndrome; and certain unusual tumors of the pituitary gland, adrenal glands, and the pancreas. Most are extremely rare, however. Hypothyroidism, which is the most common, is seldom the main reason for overweight or obesity. Treatment with thyroid hormone, while medically necessary, does not usually cause a significant weight reduction.

TRUTH

If you're overweight, it's not always your thyroid.

Hypothyroidism, the most common type of thyroid disease, affects eleven million Americans and is diagnosed through a blood test. While 15 percent of adults have thyroid issues, only 1 percent gain weight as a direct result.

Other important information your doctor will need concerns symptoms, both physical and emotional. Do you have heart disease, stroke, hypertension, or type 2 diabetes? Do you have mood swings or other symptoms of depression, such as insomnia? If so, you may need additional tests to evaluate and diagnose these problems. If you appear to have depression, anxiety, or an eating disorder, your doctor may refer you to a psychologist or psychiatrist.

Physical Exam and Screening Tests

After the medical history, you'll need a physical examination and certain screening tests. Usually, the first part of the physical exam is to measure your height and weight. This is the part we all hate, especially when the nurse instructs us to "step here on the scale first." (I always ask to take my shoes off; every ounce counts, after all.) You slip off your shoes and step gingerly onto the scale. This is one of those dreaded moments of truth. "Hmmm . . . you've gained a little extra weight," she notes. Whenever I'm asked about the 10 pounds I

TRUTH

Your "ideal weight" is the weight at which you feel your best.

There are lots of ways to measure how much you should ideally weigh, including a BMI assessment. But I feel the best measure is the weight at which you know you look good, feel good, and are at your strongest and most energetic. Maybe it's what you weighed before you had your first kid, or when you played college basketball. If you've been overweight for a very long time, even a 5 to 10 percent drop in weight will make a huge difference in how you look, feel, and move. Just be realistic. Trade in wispy dreams for a solid, livable reality.

should have lost in my thirties, I mumble, "I retain water."

Height and weight are calculated to determine your body mass index (BMI), which indicates the severity of your weight problem. Anything between 18.5 and 25 is normal; anything over 30 is obese; and everything in between is considered overweight. Your doctor should also measure the circumference of your waist and hips, since abdominal obesity increases your risk for type 2 diabetes, heart disease, and stroke. More on this fun stuff later.

A Treatment Program from Your Doctor

The plan your doctor recommends will depend on several factors, including your BMI, whether you have obesity-related health problems, and the degree of your past success in losing weight. If you are mildly overweight and in relatively good health, your doctor may be able to provide guidance on diet and exercise, have you come in for regular office visits to monitor your progress, and help you overcome the common weight-loss plateaus. Or your doctor may recommend weight-loss programs offered locally by self-help organizations, companies, registered dietitians, or hospitals. You can find a registered dietitian in your area by calling the American Dietetic Association (see Resources). By the way, your doctor has the right to know if you aren't going to follow his advice. Just say so. It is frustrating, even dangerous, for a physician to believe that you're going along with a certain regimen when you're not.

If you are extremely overweight or if you have obesity-related health problems and haven't been able to control your weight on your own, a weight-loss program that involves dieting, exercise, and social support may not be enough. In such cases, your doctor may refer you to a weight-disorders specialist or to a hospital-based

TRUTH

Focusing on numbers on your bathroom scale misses other things that count.

As the numbers on your scale begin to drop, look at other improving numbers: bringing your blood pressure, cholesterol, or blood sugar down, for example. Celebrate these improvements, because the better your numbers are, the longer you'll live.

weight-loss program. Medication and surgery are usually reserved for morbidly obese people whose weight is causing other medical problems—and who have tried everything else.

Finally, your doctor can help you set realistic goals. Most people who go through weight-loss programs lose 5 to 10 percent of their initial weight, and that's enough to lower the risk for hypertension, heart problems, diabetes—and save your life.

Yes, it's reassuring to know that your weight problem is not all your fault. And it's even better to know that you can still do a lot to get your weight under control. In light of all the factors discussed here, the attitude to have is this: Take an active role in your own weight control— through diet, exercise, better sleep, stress management, and consulting your doctor, if you need to. These actions can give you a sense of control and empowerment, and they will improve your health and longevity.

Myth #2

Your Body Shape Doesn't Matter

You don't need a medical degree to know that having high cholesterol, being a couch potato, and smoking are bad for your body. But in recent years, other surprising factors have popped up that can put your health at risk. Among them: a chubby waistline.

When I lived in San Francisco, I had a neighbor, Ellen McCall, a forty-one-year-old mother of three. She had been battling her weight for years and was particularly heavy around her waist, but that was just one health issue plaguing her. Ellen had a family history of high cholesterol but considered herself far too young to worry about it. Then, for several weeks in 1997, Ellen had been feeling unusually tired, suffering from nasty bouts of heartburn and stomach pain. But the stay-at-home mom chalked up her symptoms to stress. "I am so busy raising these three little boys, I'm sure the craziness of my schedule is at least partly to blame," she told me.

So when Ellen awoke at 3 o'clock one summer morning, feeling as if her windpipe was being clawed out of her chest, she assumed she had eaten too much rich food and was suffering from heartburn again. Ellen headed to the bathroom for her heartburn medicine. Never once did she think she might be having a heart attack.

Minutes later, her husband found Ellen collapsed on the bathroom floor. Horrified, he called 911. Although paramedics worked frantically to save her, Ellen had suffered a full-blown heart attack, and she was dead. Only after she died were we able to piece together her heart disease history and look at all the risk factors that we never knew about.

A growing number of women are losing their lives to heart disease. Already, one in three women in the United States has cardiovascular disease, and more than 460,000 women die of heart disease every year. Hundreds of thousands more may be at risk. Yet many physicians continue to pay less attention to risk factors in women than in men.

We all know the stereotypical picture of a heart attack seen on TV and in the movies: People clutch their chest and fall dramatically to the floor. But for real-life women, chest pain may not be the most prominent symptom—or even a symptom at all. Heart attacks often start with only mild chest discomfort—hours, days, or even weeks before the actual event. Other symptoms include pressure in the chest; radiating pain to the limbs, shoulders, neck, or back; stomach upset; overwhelming fatigue; sweats; dizziness; or fainting. Any one of these could be a sign of an impending heart attack. Far too many women don't recognize that these symptoms are warnings.

But here's something that does serve as a warning flag: your body shape. Men and women with large waists, regardless of body size, are more likely to have risk factors for heart disease than those who are overweight or obese all over. In Ellen's case, she probably suffered from something doctors call metabolic syndrome, a cluster of symptoms that include a large waistline, higher-than-normal blood pressure, unhealthy cholesterol levels, elevated triglycerides, and high blood sugar. The more of these factors you have, the more likely you will develop heart disease, diabetes, or stroke. In fact, a person with metabolic syndrome is twice as likely to develop heart disease, and five times as likely to develop diabetes, as someone without the condition, says the National Institutes of Health. And by the way, metabolic syndrome carries a worse prognosis for women than men. The reason is unclear; however, it may be related to emotions. Depression and stressful life events—experienced by women more than by men—are risk factors for metabolic syndrome.

So does body shape matter? You bet it does. And your life may just depend on it.

THE SHAPE OF YOUR HEALTH

Have those "love handles" made it hard to tie your shoes? Does your belt need a new hole—or two or three? And what's going on with your jeans? Why is everything so darn tight around your thighs?

If you find yourself asking these questions while you try to pull that zipper all the way up, join the club. Our national paunch is expanding—a lot. The average American waistline has never been bigger. Federal health surveys show that over the past four decades, the average waist size for men has grown from 35 inches to 39 inches; for women, from 30 inches to 37 inches. This isn't a good omen for our health. Medical researchers now say, the bigger your waist, the unhealthier your life.

Once considered an old wives' tale, it has now been proven that body shape can be an indicator of an increased risk of serious diseases. Fat around the waist, for example, has been linked to not only a greater risk of heart disease, diabetes, and stroke but also hypertension, breathing problems, disability, some cancers, and higher mortality rates overall.

TRUTH

The average American gains less than a pound during the holidays.

The gain is a mere 0.8 pound, to be exact. It's a myth that we pack on 5 to 10 pounds during the food-filled six weeks between Thanksgiving and New Year's. But while we might not gain that much weight, we forget to take it off in the spring. Those ounces accumulate incrementally, year after year, and we don't notice until we try to jimmy into what used to be our fat jeans. Strategy: Monitor your weight in the winter. If it's up, act quickly with exercise and diet to take it off. It's a lot easier to lose a pound or so today than 20 pounds later.

ANATOMY OF A MYTH

Blame this myth on us doctors. The medical community once believed that it was weight itself or a high body mass index, a measure of overall fatness based on your height, which led to serious illness and earlier death, not where the fat is located on the body. But recent research on the workings of the fat cell has shown that not all fat is alike and has different "weight" depending on where it is deposited on the body. Tummy fat is dangerous, while hip and thigh fat is more benign.

For years, many doctors and scientists have divided overweight people into two groups, according to body shape: apples and pears. Apple-shaped people carry much of their fat above the waist, while pear-shaped people

TRUTH

Low-calorie diets may shrink your stomach.

When researchers at Columbia University's Obesity Research Center in New York put obese patients on a 600-calorie-a-day diet for four weeks, the dieters' stomach capacities were reduced by 27 percent, so they reported feeling more satisfied with fewer calories. The researchers believe these findings may also apply to the average dieter, giving credence to the fact that you can indeed "shrink your stomach." One caveat: I don't recommend going as low as 600 calories a day, however; that's too low and can backfire. It may cause your body to believe it's starving and alter your metabolic rate. Depriving yourself also may lead to bingeing and overeating. It's better to make smaller changes and cut 250 to 500 calories from your usual daily intake.

carry much of their fat on hips and thighs. Men tend to be apples and women pears, largely because of hormonal differences.

Which shape are you? Here's how to easily figure it out if you're not sure: First thing in the morning, take your waist (level with your belly button) and hip measurements (around the widest part of hips and buttocks) in inches. Divide your waist measurement by your hip measurement. If the result is less than 0.8, this is a pear shape. If the figure is above 0.8, this is an apple shape.

Apples: The Belly Burden

Apple bears the classic appearance of the middle-age spread, with weight around the stomach giving a barrel-like tummy and narrow hips. An apple body shape—also known as an "android type"—occurs when higher levels of testosterone in the body cause fat to be stored around the stomach. It is actually more typical of men, which explains why they're more prone to beer bellies.

This belly fat is hyperactive, meaning it breaks down and enters the bloodstream readily. This was great in prehistoric times when a man's body required ready supplies of quick-release fat to hunt animals for food. But since the only hunting some men do for food in modern times is hunting down a beer in the fridge, that same fat is more likely to be absorbed into the bloodstream, where it can raise cholesterol levels and lead to clogged arteries, high blood pressure, and other problems.

When fat accumulates in the stomach and waist area, it doesn't just build up under the skin, it also builds up inside the upper torso and gathers around the heart, liver, kidneys, and intestines. Some experts believe it can even begin to grow inside these organs, restricting blood flow and interfering with their function.

Fat around the middle is largely visceral fat, a type of deep fat that drapes itself around internal organs and spews hormones and other chemicals, some of them harmful or inflammatory. One, for instance, is tumor necrosis factor-alpha, which can trigger insulin resistance. Visceral fat sets off reactions in the body that lead to changes in arteries, organs, and cells that result in heart disease, diabetes, and probably some cancers. The more abdominal fat, the greater the risk of developing these conditions earlier. Visceral fat is toxic fat.

Studies also show that fat cells in the abdomen have a much greater influence on the hormone insulin than fat elsewhere. This means apples are more prone to diabetes.

Apple-shaped women have higher rates of breast cancer. Although the exact relationship isn't clear, one theory is that fat tissue stores estrogen—a hormone known to influence breast cancer. It may be that the more estrogen stored around your stomach and upper body, the higher your risk of the disease. Plus, some experts believe the excess insulin produced by women with abdominal fat could raise levels of insulin-like growth factor, high levels of which have been linked to breast tumors.

Are you at risk for any of these health problems? Studies suggest that health risks begin to increase when a woman's waist reaches 31.5 inches, and her risk jumps substantially once her waist expands to 35 inches or more. For a man, risk starts to climb at 37 inches, but it

TRUTH

Belly fat is linked with dementia.

Here's yet another reason for getting rid of that big belly. People who have large stomachs in their forties are at greater risk of developing dementia when they reach their seventies, says a 2008 study published in *Neurology*. The study stops short of proving that belly fat causes dementia, but it does suggest a connection between the two. Those who were overweight and had a large belly were 2.3 times more likely to develop dementia than those with a normal weight and belly size. Those who were obese and had a large belly were 3.6 times more likely to develop dementia.

becomes a bigger worry once his waist reaches or exceeds 40 inches.

One easy way to keep tabs on your risk is to measure your waist periodically. Then compare it with your height. If the circumference of your waist is less than half your height, you don't need to worry.

Pears: Fat Chance

Being pear shaped may be a lot healthier than being apple shaped. The fat cells on the thighs and hips tend to break down slowly and are less likely to travel around the body and do damage. The pear shape is the traditional female shape because a woman's body is primed to need fat that is slow burning, like thigh and hip fat, to provide enough energy for pregnancy and breast-feeding.

I have three children and fed each one a different way. Kate, my oldest, is adopted and was thus bottle fed.

TRUTH

Monounsaturated fats may help flatten your tummy.

I've always had a love affair with olive oil. I love the taste, and since it is an unsaturated fat it may play an ongoing role in keeping my low-density lipoprotein (LDL, or "bad cholesterol") in check. Because it's so flavorful, I use it for practically everything—from salads to stir-fries. Now there's a reason for me to love it even more: A 2006 study published in *Diabetes Care* reported that monounsaturated fats like olive oil may help prevent body fat from accumulating around the stomach. These fats appear to help your body use insulin better and have positive effects on other hormones involved in weight control. Monounsaturated fats also come from avocados as well as canola and peanut oils.

My second and third children were breast fed. One of the many benefits of breast-feeding is that it is one of the few ways of reducing a big thigh measurement. I can attest to that. My thighs slimmed down after months of feeding my babies. I'm not alone. Many women report the same kind of changes after breast-feeding.

Hip and thigh fat may actually offer some unique safeguard against cardiovascular disease, particularly for women. Women with larger hips and more weight on their bottom and thighs are less likely to suffer heart attacks, angina, diabetes, high blood pressure, or cardiovascular disease.

But not all researchers agree that hip fat is beneficial, since more lower-body fat generally means more fat—period—which can lead to higher risk of heart disease and diabetes. And although heart conditions and strokes are rarer among pear shapes, they are more prone to ovarian cancer, breast cysts, and endometriosis. But with diet, exercise, and proper care, your pear shape can vanish, taking with it the increased risks of these health issues.

WHAT TO DO ABOUT THE SHAPE YOU'RE IN

So what can you do if you're shaped more like an apple than a pear? And if you don't like being a pear, can you downsize your thighs? While genetics play a major role in body shape, you can do something about your shape. Knowing your body shape measurements gives you a head start in protecting yourself and helps you reverse the course of diseases through diet, exercise, and other lifestyle changes. Here's how you can keep your shape in shape.

Know Your Family History

Look to your family tree to see how far your apple shape has fallen from that tree. Your family history adds to your risk of developing heart disease. If you have a family history of heart disease, you are at risk for heart disease. If your father had a heart attack before the age of fifty-six or if your mother had one before the age of sixty, you are considered at risk for heart disease—so you should take precautions. Losing even as few as 10 pounds can lower your heart disease risk. You can further reduce your risk by altering your body-fat distribution, using the suggestions that follow.

Talk About Body Shape at Your Next Doctor's Visit

Discuss your body shape during your next visit to your physician. If your waist–hip measurement is in the critical zone, you'll have to be vigilant. Treat your body shape as a warning sign and an impetus to change bad habits. If you are overweight or obese, begin a weight-loss program. (Don't beat yourself up to get overnight results. Weight goes on gradually, and if you do it the right way, it comes off gradually and stays off longer.) If these methods don't seem to be enough, you may want to discuss medication with your doctor as a last resort. If your cholesterol, triglycerides, or blood pressure is elevated, lower the fat content of your diet, eat more fiber and complex carbohydrates, and cut back on red meats.

TRUTH

Liposuction can recontour your shape but it doesn't reduce health risks.

Many people are tempted by the notion of sucking out those excess pounds from their hips or other paunchy areas. And it is effective for removing diet- and exercise-resistant fat deposits, especially when used on the lower abdomen, buttocks, and thighs. But while liposuction helps you get rid of visible fat, health risks remain. In a study in the *New England Journal of Medicine,* fifteen obese women lost an average of 23 pounds through liposuction, but tests measuring insulin resistance, blood pressure, and blood levels of cholesterol, triglycerides, and other substances used to gauge heart-disease and diabetes risk showed no changes after the procedure. Losing weight through diet and exercise, however, does reduce those risks.

Make Exercise a Part of Your Life

Exercise is a great way to do some shape shifting. Apples, you'll find it easier to drop excess weight than pears, because abdominal fat breaks down much faster than fat around the hips. In fact, it's the first to disappear when you exercise. By exercising and losing excess stomach fat, apples will reduce their risk of disease. Aerobic exercise (running, swimming, cycling) will help to reduce the layer of fat apples are prone to. Combining free weights with squats, lunges, and twists will work your waist muscles, toning them but not spot reducing the fat. With a combination of aerobics, weight training, and proper diet, your abdominal fat will diminish—and your risk for heart disease will, too.

Pears can cut their chance of suffering from disease, too. Aim to reduce fat on your hips and thighs with diet

EXTRA, EXTRA

Strength training prevents middle-aged spread.

Beginning in your midtwenties, belly fat begins to creep on by a pound or two a year—a jeans-zipping challenge and, more seriously, a health concern. But you can slow the spread with strength training. In a study at the University of Minnesota, overweight women who lifted weights just twice a week saw a much smaller increase in abdominal fat (7 percent) over a two-year period than women who didn't follow any particular exercise program (theirs went up 21 percent). Strength training doesn't take the place of a cardio workout, but it's an effective way to keep your waist trim if practiced only two days a week.

and exercise. Let aerobic exercise take care of fat burning. Running is great for pears, but cycling should be avoided, as it can bulk up your legs.

Check Out the "Apple Diet"

In 2007 a study published in the *Journal of the American Medical Association* caught my eye. It revealed that certain dieters, those who get a hefty surge of the hormone insulin every time they eat a doughnut or hot-fudge sundae, lose more weight on diets with fewer carbohydrates and more fat. Those who churn out less insulin don't get the same benefits. It is believed that perhaps apple-shaped people tend to secrete higher amounts of insulin compared with pear shapes.

In this study, researchers measured the insulin levels of seventy-three obese adults, without diabetes, after they drank a sugary beverage. One group was told to follow a "low-glycemic diet" of fruits, vegetables, and barley, with carb intake cut to no more than 40 percent of calories. (A low-glycemic diet includes foods designed to keep blood sugar on an even keel. This type of diet is different from a low-carb diet, which typically eliminates foods like barley and fruit.) A second group could eat a variety of carbs but had to restrict fat intake to 20 percent of their calories.

After eighteen months, dieters who had the highest insulin spikes at the beginning of the study had lost nearly 13 pounds on the low-glycemic diet; their counterparts on a low-fat diet shed an average of just 3 pounds. The low insulin makers in the study lost the same 3 pounds even when they were put on the low-glycemic diet. Both diets cut daily food intake by 400 calories.

What explains the different diet outcomes? The researchers speculated that most high insulin secretors have probably been following a low-fat, high-carb diet for years, so they packed on extra weight that easily came off once they lowered insulin levels.

If you've been having trouble losing weight, it may not be a bad idea to find out if your body is churning out a lot of insulin. A routine glucose tolerance blood test that involves drinking a sugar solution and having a blood sample drawn thirty minutes later will yield the answer. Or, if you don't want to go to the trouble, tinker a bit with your eating plan to see if going on a lower-carb or lower-glycemic diet helps.

TRUTH

Mesotherapy is an unproven fat fix.

One of the latest body-sculpting trends to hit the United States is mesotherapy. It's a controversial procedure in which doctors use tiny needles to inject a variety of ingredients, including heart and arthritis drugs, plant extracts, hormones, and enzymes, into the mesoderm—the layers of fat and connective tissue under the skin. Mesotherapy promises to "melt" fat by breaking up fat cells, releasing them into the bloodstream where they are somehow metabolized. The procedure is not approved by the U.S. Food and Drug Administration, and recent studies have not been able to prove that it is effective for body contouring.

If You Smoke, Stop

Contrary to what many dieters think, one of the worst things for your waist—and the worst thing for your health—is cigarettes. Smokers tend to store fat around the waist and upper torso. That's the conclusion of a growing and compelling amount of research into the relationship between fat distribution and smoking. One large-scale study, in particular, analyzed data from 21,828 men and women who were forty-five to seventy-nine years of age and found that the smokers tended to be chubby around the waist. In another study of nearly twelve thousand premenopausal and postmenopausal women ages forty to seventy-three, the women's waistline increased as the number of cigarettes smoked per day increased.

What's the connection? By throwing your endocrine system out of whack (glands that secrete hormones), smoking affects fat distribution by causing fat to be stored centrally—around the middle. Of course, these changes to your waistline don't have to be permanent. If you stop smoking, less fat will collect around your waist. So is smoking cessation a way to influence and control your body shape? Absolutely!

Cigarette smoking is a powerful addiction, and it can be tremendously difficult to give up. Here's some help for the journey:

- Get support. Tell your friends and family of your plans.
- Set a date when you will quit.

- Pick your method: cold turkey, antidepressants, and/or over-the-counter medications such as nicotine replacements (nicotine gum or nicotine patches).
- Change your daily routine as much as is possible to avoid situations that encourage you to smoke, including triggers such as hanging out with friends who smoke, or drinking alcohol.
- Don't frequent places that encourage you to smoke, such as bars, and avoid parties. Fortunately, many bars these days are smoke-free.
- Engage in other activities when the urge to smoke hits: go for a walk, chew gum, take a shower (it's tough to smoke while you're showering), or call a friend for support.
- If you have trouble quitting, consult your doctor regarding smoking-cessation drugs that can help you kick the chemical addiction.
- Find a support group and keep trying.
- Don't assume it's hopeless if you go back to smoking after quitting. The odds are actually better that you will quit for good if you have quit once or twice before.
- Most important, never give up, ever!

Curb Cocktails

One of the obvious effects of drinking too much alcohol is a beer belly. When you drink alcohol, your body burns up fat more slowly than usual, not to mention that alcohol also increases your appetite. Any fat that is not burned will be stored, and excess calories from alcohol tend to congregate at the midsection at a faster rate than others, most likely because alcohol may affect metabolic processes in the liver.

Alcohol can be a part of a weight-loss plan, as long as you count its calories into your daily allotment and consider a cocktail as a treat. Moderate drinking does not seem to increase abdominal fat, but having four or more drinks in one sitting does. So avoid excessive drinking, or binge drinking, or else you risk getting fat around your middle.

If you think you need to cut down on alcohol, what can you do? Greater awareness of how much of the stuff we're putting away would be a good place to start. If you have a drink, drink it slowly. Keep within the limits of moderation, if you drink at all: No more than two drinks a day for men; no more than one a day for women. If you don't want the calories, try something I do: have a glass of club soda with lime. It's calorie-free.

We still have a lot to learn about body shape, waist size, and metabolism. The best thing to do for now is to stop waist expansion and slow down the process of becoming more applelike. Take a bite out of this apple: it really does matter.

Myth #3

Calories Don't Count

I got fat, and it wasn't hard to figure out why.

Remember the "freshman 15," those insidious, unwanted pounds that college students (particularly women) tend to gain during that first year of college? Like many of the other girls on my dorm floor, I gained the freshman 15, but they quickly became the freshman 30. In the seventies, dormitories didn't serve food as some do now. We were left on our own. And I splurged on pizza, strombolis, boxes of cookies, bags of chips, and beer. I ate when I was happy; I ate when I was sad. I ate when I was hungry; I ate when I wasn't hungry. I loved fast food so much I even considered working at a hamburger joint so I could get the employee discount and eat all I wanted.

It's an understatement that college is an academically challenging time for transition and transformation. It also meant leaving the nest, leaving behind the cooking

I'd been familiar with for eighteen years. It was my first shot at independence, a time to become my own person. Being in college brought a new freedom to eat whatever I pleased, whenever I wanted it.

I also entered college at a time of social upheaval, and I abandoned the sports I had grown up with. I ditched tennis and swimming and made the error of not replacing those activities with anything, except for walking to class. Combined with my nonstop appetite, being sedentary put me in pound-packing peril.

I eventually tipped the scales at 200 pounds. I was so self-conscious about how I looked that rather than walking through the main doors of the amphitheater where lectures were given, I slipped through the doors at the top so no one could see me. I felt so unattractive that I kept to myself and concentrated on following the family tradition of becoming a doctor. It was a sad time for me, and getting fat just made it worse. I wrapped the fat around me like a protective blanket. My fat was an unconscious statement, a metaphor, about how I wanted to insulate myself from life.

My first time home after gaining so much weight, my family barely recognized me. I'll never forget the day my brother asked, "What happened to you?"

As I sat down on my bed one day, hating the way my belt cut into my waist, I knew I had to do something. I was miserable and my self-esteem was in the toilet. I had to lose weight or go out and buy a whole new wardrobe (of which I was sure my parents wouldn't approve). This began my search for the perfect weight-loss plan, a search that had nothing to do with health but began instead out of desperation over my ballooning weight. Over the next few months I experimented with different fad diets, but nothing really worked for long.

I got so depressed over the ups and downs in my weight that I ate to assuage my depression. For those who've never done it, it sounds crazy, I know, but those who have been there know exactly how I felt. And it was such a vicious cycle. I ate because I was depressed and I was depressed because I ate.

After years of this misery, I had had about all I could take of being fat and depressed about it. (When you start getting on your own nerves, you know you have a problem.) I was ready to make major lifestyle changes to feel better about myself, mentally and physically. I wanted to feel comfortable in my own skin—something I had not been in a long time. A friend suggested that I see a therapist to deal with my weight and emotional eating issues. I thought it was a dumb idea, since therapy to me was a sign that you couldn't manage things on your own. But I did it anyway, since I had no other options.

In therapy, I began to listen to myself, hear my words, and recognize parts of me that were valuable and worthy. I began to realize that filling up with food was a way to fill a void in my life. Permanent weight loss would be impossible until I figured out who I was and learned to find other nonfood ways to deal with my feelings. My therapist encouraged me to meditate, a practice I still consider valuable, though I struggle with it at times. Those quiet times of solitary thought provide moments of renewal.

Bit by bit, I began to heal. Although I still consider

myself a work in progress, I learned to lay the foundation for a healthier life, in much the same way I was laying a foundation for my medical career. The emotional eating, having served its purpose, stopped, and my weight drifted back to a normal, healthy 140, give or take a few pounds.

That's not to say I haven't struggled with my weight since college. Every day, I am thankful for my body because, while I have some good and bad days, it has never betrayed me. Some days, I'm good; some days, I slip. Some days, I really care; some days, I don't care so much. But there is one thing I do consistently: count calories.

Yes, count calories! Maybe you've heard that calories don't count. Ha! Here I'll bust the biggest diet myth of

TRUTH

Yo-yo dieting won't wreck your metabolism.

Because of all the ups and downs I've experienced with my weight through the years, I was afraid that dieting might have messed with my metabolism. Now I've learned I don't have anything to worry about. While extremely low-cal diets temporarily lower your metabolism, recent studies suggest that the effects don't last. Researchers in Canada looked at fifty-two overweight women who'd been dieting on and off for an average of eighteen years. They measured the women's resting metabolic rate, then compared those numbers with what their metabolism was expected to be based on their weights, heights, and ages. The result: There was no difference between actual and predicted metabolic rates in all but four dieters. So even if you've lost and regained weight countless times, don't give up. Yo-yo diets don't hurt you; they just don't get you anywhere.

all—as well as tell you why weight-loss experts are now advocating the back-to-basics approach of calorie counting.

ANATOMY OF A MYTH

So where did the whole calories-don't-count myth originate? It's hard to say for sure, but some experts trace it to the title of a 1961 diet book called *Calories Don't Count* by Romanian-born gynecologist Dr. Herman Taller. His title introduced into popular vernacular a phrase that continues to haunt us to this very day. Naturally, it was one many dieters wanted to hear, and two million of them rushed out to buy it. Taller's diet was of the low-carb variety and encouraged dieters to eat large quantities of unsaturated vegetable fat. In 1967 Taller was convicted

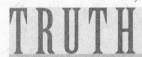

Slashing as many calories as possible is not a good way to lose weight.

At first blush, it might seem logical to cut as many calories as you can to make the pounds drop off fast. But this mind-set often backfires. You feel hungry, deprived, and ready to gorge. It's consistency that gets you to your goal: eating less in the long run and burning more. To do this, reduce your calories slowly. Your body will recognize this as a gradual reduction. It will not revolt because it thinks you are in starvation mode. Slash your calories in half or more, and your body will register this as a shock and hold on to the pounds—not what you want.

of mail fraud for selling "worthless" safflower oil capsules as supplements.

Dieters continued disregarding calories even when low-fat, high-carbohydrate diets became the rage. Millions were led to believe by health authorities that *all* dietary fat was the true cause of obesity (another myth). Cutting fat and replacing it with carbohydrate was the key to getting slim, these diets claimed, and everyone started counting fat grams rather than counting calories. Ironically, the original reasoning given for this claim was fat was a high-calorie item. Each gram of fat contains 9 calories; by contrast a gram of carbohydrate is 4 calories and a gram of protein is 4 calories. This means that gram for gram fat contains two and a quarter times more calories than carbs or protein.

TRUTH

Dark chocolate is a dieter's friend.

Dark chocolate is not your average sweet. It contains a natural compound that makes blood platelets less likely to stick together and cause abnormal clots. This helps blood flow, promotes normal clotting, and improves circulation. The darker the chocolate, the healthier it is. Sure, eating pounds and pounds of chocolate will pack on the pounds, but that's not what I'm talking about. It can be incorporated in your diet, as long as you enjoy it in moderation. A one-ounce serving counts as "moderate" and contains around 110 calories. My friend Dr. Susan Love loves her chocolate so much that she says, laughing, it should be its own food group. Look for chocolate with at least 70 percent cocoa in it for the best benefit—and enjoy a little every now and then.

As dieters got disillusioned with low-fat dieting, they increasingly turned toward its polar opposite: the low-carbohydrate diet. Beginning in the late 1990s, a string of best-selling low-carbohydrate diet books began hitting the shelves. A common theme among these authors was that a high-protein, high-fat diet allowed you to eat all you wanted without putting on pounds. The true culprit of weight gain, claimed these authors, was carbohydrates. Readers were urged to forget about counting calories and instead focus on cutting carbohydrates while enjoying all sorts of fats, including artery-clogging saturated fats. The concept of consuming lots of saturated fats, without regard for balance, has just never made sense to me.

So low-carb, high-carb, low-fat, or high-protein? It doesn't matter, according to a Harvard study published in the February 26, 2009, issue of *The New England Journal of Medicine*. Researchers assigned 811 overweight adults

TRUTH

Dessert can be dinner.

Don't call the food police on me for this one, but I say you can enjoy a Rocky Road ice-cream dinner "now and then," which means as an occasional deal and not a steady routine. Don't deny yourself certain cravings. Make a meal out of a favorite treat and you'll be less tempted to overindulge on your splurge foods. Just swap the steak out for the sundae and know that this tactic is for the occasional treat, not the everyday occurrence—and it may help you be more successful in controlling your weight over the long term.

to one of four diets, each of which contained different amounts of fat, protein, and carbs. No matter which approach was used, the food plans cut about 750 calories from the diet. Everyone lost an average of 13 pounds after six months, and kept off 9 pounds after two years, regardless of which diet they followed. The "magic formula" to weight loss isn't about gimmicky diets. It's about calories in, calories out.

WHAT EXACTLY IS A CALORIE, ANYWAY?

You can't have been on any diet without having the word *calorie* driven into your consciousness. As much as many diets would have you think otherwise, and as much as you may want to hear otherwise, losing weight boils down to a simple formula: Eat fewer calories than you burn. Break that rule and all the carb-cutting, fat-banning, low-glycemic-index eating in the world won't make a bit of difference. And if one diet promises that you can consume lots of calories and still lose weight, it's lying to you.

But do you know what a calorie really is? It's a measure of potential energy in food. Technically, 1 calorie is the amount of energy it takes to raise the temperature of 1 gram of water by 1 degree Celsius.

Your body converts calories into energy. During the digestion and absorption of food in your intestine, enzymes break the chemical bonds that hold food molecules together. The energy contained in those bonds is released, making it available for use. That energy fuels everything from basic activities like breathing, thinking, and growing hair to bigger tasks, like being pregnant or running a marathon.

When you don't use the calories you've consumed (maybe you decide to skip your workout today), those

TRUTH

Salads can fatten you up.

Want to see the perfect recipe for getting fat? Watch people at a salad bar. Everyone knows that lettuce and raw veggies are indeed low in calories, but glob on only two tablespoons of dressing and you've added more than 200 calories to your salad. Chef salads consist of about 5 ounces of roast beef, hard cheese, ham, hard-boiled egg—that's nearly 400 calories of animal protein. (For an alternative, try grilled chicken on a bed of mixed greens, with dressing on the side.) Caesar salads can run as high as 900 calories or more. Also, premixed salad with a mayonnaise base is a disaster in the making. Keep your salads and dressings simple. Get the taste of your favorite dressing by having it served on the side, dipping your fork into the dressing, then spearing your salad. Better yet, splash on balsamic vinegar with some herbs. Yummy!

TRUTH

Salads can slim you down.

Yes, you read that right, and I'm not trying to contradict myself or confuse you. Here's how you can use a salad to slim you down: Eat a large salad of greens and salad veggies (dressing on the side) prior to your main course. It will make you feel full, and you'll eat less at your meal.

calories get shuttled to your liver to refill your glycogen stores. Glycogen, which is stored carbohydrate obtained from food, is your body's quick, easy-access energy reserve. Because your body can store it, you don't have to eat continuously to keep your body revved up. Still, it gets depleted every three to four hours, and this triggers hunger. When the liver is holding as much glycogen as it can, some of it is passed on to muscles for short-term storage (to be used as needed to move your body or get you through a workout).

So between your liver and muscles, you have a ready tank of calories (roughly 300 to 400, depending on your weight and metabolism) that you can access as needed throughout the day. And that's where the equation takes a big right turn. When you eat more than can be deposited

TRUTH

Calorie-free soft drinks may make you fat.

I've never been a big fan of diet drinks (I prefer good old water), and now I'm glad. A study conducted by the University of Texas Health Science Center at San Antonio followed over six hundred people ranging from twenty-five to sixty-four years old for up to eight years and found that those drinking diet soda—even as little as one can or bottle a day—did not lose weight and were significantly more likely to become overweight than those who drank regular soft drinks or none at all. How can this be? No one knows for sure, but scientists think that artificial sweeteners, perhaps even the caramel coloring, may muddle brain chemistry. The brain in a sense gets a reward, and the desire for more sweets is intensified. The more of these fake sweet products you eat or drink, the more sweets you want.

in the liver and muscles, the calories have to go somewhere so they get converted to fat and are deposited as body fat on your hips, thighs, belly, and elsewhere. And once they set up shop there, it can be tough to turn and get back on track with weight control.

CALORIES: HOW MUCH?

Think of your body as a bank account—I consider it my "energy account"—in which I make energy deposits (by eating calories) and energy withdrawals (by burning calories through exercise). Like my bank account, if I put in more than I take out, the balance grows. This notion is what dietitians call energy balance, and it has three important components: When calorie intake equals calories burned, you are in energy balance, a steady state, and maintaining your weight. When calorie intake is greater than calories burned, you are in a positive energy balance and gaining weight. When calorie intake is less than energy burned, you are in negative energy balance and losing weight.

While I measure my bank account in dollars, my energy account is measured in calories. It takes about 3,500 calories to equal a pound on the scale. Every time my energy account balance increases by 3,500 calories, I gain about a pound. Every time my energy account balance decreases by 3,500 calories, I lose about a pound. For managing weight, the key question we all need to ask is: How many calories do I need to lose, maintain, or gain weight?

To be really accurate, you'll want to know what your "basal metabolic rate"—otherwise known as your BMR—is for someone of your height, weight, and sex. Your BMR is the rate at which you burn calories at rest just to maintain vital body functions, such as breathing and heartbeat and brain activity, among others. Your BMR usually accounts for at least half of the calories you burn in a day. There's a formula for figuring this out, and it depends on your age, sex, and level of daily physical activity. It's a little complicated, but if you like to crunch numbers I've provided it for you in the chart on page 66. If you'd rather not do the math, several websites can calculate your BMR. Just complete the formula by filling in your height, weight, and age, and your BMR will be estimated. Try the BMR calculators on the following websites: www.bmi-calculator.net/bmr-calculator or www.womenfitness.net/bmr.htm.

Now here's the burning question: Once you've figured out how many calories you need to maintain your current weight, how many calories should you cut if you want to lose weight?

Remember, to lose just 1 pound, you must burn 3,500 calories. If you want to lose 1 to 2 pounds a week—a safe rate of weight loss—you can reach that goal by decreasing the calories you eat or increasing the calories you burn by 250 to 500 calories a day, depending on your current caloric intake. (By the same token, you can gain weight by eating 250 to 500 calories more a day.)

Before you yawn, here's the advantage: the weight you take off slowly is the weight that stays off longest.

How to Figure Your Metabolic Rate

For women:

$655 + (4.36 \times your\ weight\ in\ pounds) + (4.32 \times your\ height\ in\ inches) - (4.7 \times your\ age) = BMR$

I did the math for a thirty-year-old woman who is 5 foot 6 inches tall and weighs 140 pounds.

$BMR\ (equals)\ 655 + 609 + 310.2 - 141.$ Her BMR is 1433.2.

For men:

$66 + (6.22 \times your\ weight\ in\ pounds) + (12.7 \times your\ height\ in\ inches) - (6.8 \times your\ age) = BMR$

I did the calculations for a thirty-year-old man who is 6 feet tall and weighs 175 pounds.

$BMR\ (equals)\ 66 + 1090.25 + 914.4 - 204.$ His BMR is 1866.65.

Once you know your BMR, factor in your activity level to figure out the exact calories you need daily to maintain your weight.

1. If you are sedentary (little or no exercise), you multiply your BMR by 1.2.
2. If you are lightly active (light exercise/sports 1 to 3 days/week), you multiply your BMR by 1.375.
3. If you are moderately active (moderate exercise/sports 3 to 5 days/week), you multiply your BMR by 1.55.
4. If you are very active (hard exercise/sports 6 to 7 days a week), you multiply your BMR by 1.725.
5. If you are extra active (very hard exercise/sports plus a physical job or training twice a day), you multiply your BMR by 1.9.

This approach works, and it's a long-term deal. If you do it right and do it once, you can reclaim your life and not be a slave to constant dieting.

Bottom line, there's only one way to lose weight, and it's inherently boring and not at all glamorous: Burn off

TRUTH

Fasting undermines weight loss.

Proponents of fasting say it's a good way to give your body's digestive system a break or jump-start weight loss. Not true. Neither the human body nor the digestive system need breaks, only well-spaced rest periods between meals. Your entire body was designed to be on the job around the clock. When you go on a fast of eating nothing, your body thinks it's starving. It does everything it can to protect you and starts to conserve fat and calories. In starvation mode, your metabolic rate slows down, and muscle tissue gets burned preferentially over fat. You burn very little fat on a fast. While fasting, you feel pretty yucky, too. Who needs that?

more calories than you take in. The only time calories don't count, as far as I'm concerned, is on vacation or holidays and on my birthday. After all, having fun in life does involve some rule breaking.

IS A CALORIE A CALORIE . . . ?

Are some calories more fattening than others? Are the calories you get from eating carbs worse than the calories from fats? Or is it the other way around?

The confusion comes about because the body processes carbohydrates, protein, and fat differently. Simple carbohydrates, such as sugar and white bread, break down fast in the body and are absorbed quickly. On the other hand, complex carbohydrates (like beans) take longer to digest, as do protein and fat.

The answer: You can eat 200 carbohydrate calories

and lay down the same amount of fat as if you ate 200 fat calories. If you want to lose or maintain weight, you can juggle the proportion of fat, carbohydrates, and protein in your diet, but the total number of calories you take in still counts. There's a catch, however, and it depends on the quality of what you eat. You get more nutrient bang for those 200 calories if they come from carbs like fresh fruits and vegetables than if you ate 200 calories of pure fat.

The overwhelming amount of evidence for this includes a paper published in 1992 in the *American Journal of Clinical Nutrition* by researchers at Rockefeller Univer-

TRUTH

Liquid calories count.

If and when you tally up your calories at the end of a meal or a day, do your calculations take into account what you drank? Do you remember to include that can of soda, smoothie, cup of latte, or cocktail? People tend to guzzle their calories and it really adds up, often more than they realize. For example, that can of soda you drink each morning is the calorie equivalent of a piece of fruit and a slice of toast, about 150 calories. A smoothie can run up to an extra 500 to 1,000 calories despite all the good stuff added in, and a 16-ounce latte with whole milk packs 260 calories. The average margarita—my favorite—has more than 500 calories. What's more, the brain doesn't seem to register liquid calories as accurately as calories that are chewed, and it doesn't send stop-eating signals to keep you from eating more food. If you're taking in only 1,200 to 1,500 calories a day, save those calories for food. Liquid calories add up quickly, so stick with water and calorie-free beverages, and you could lose a pound or more a week. I lost 5 pounds last month because I decided not to have a cocktail periodically with friends.

sity. The authors put people on a metabolic ward where they could precisely control every calorie consumed. The subjects were on widely varied diets for thirty-three days, with widely different compositions of nutrients. The source of the calories they ate made no difference in how much weight the people gained or lost. All that mattered to their weight was the number of calories consumed. In April 2001 the *Journal of the American Dietetic Association* reviewed two hundred studies that looked at nutrient composition of diets and weight loss. Conclusion: "Weight loss is independent of diet composition."

Alas, there is no metabolic magic to any particular popular diet to make you gain or lose weight. What ultimately matters for weight control are calories. It makes no difference if those calories are in fats or vegetables or cake or ice cream or rib-eyes, except when it comes to nutritional value.

The quality of your diet definitely matters. You need to eat a variety of foods and get your calories from many

TRUTH

Eating fat won't make you fat.

Plenty of thin people eat fat! They eat fat, but they just don't overindulge on calories. So scratch the "eat fat, get fat" theory and start counting calories instead. There, I've said it again: eat too many calories, and don't be surprised if the scale goes up. On the other hand, if you cut back on fatty foods, you will lose body fat by creating a calorie deficit. You need a little fat for good health; plus, it adds satiety—the nice feeling of being satisfied after a meal.

sources. Of the three ways to take in a calorie—proteins, carbohydrates, and fats—your body needs all three in sensible amounts. Any program or diet that eliminates or severely limits any of these macronutrients isn't sustainable, nor is it healthy. If your calories aren't from nutritious food, you may be thin, but you won't feel or look your best. There is a scientific rhyme and reason to food, and once understood, your nutritional choices become easier and the road to health and proper weight a reality. For instance, carbohydrates like whole grains, vegetables, and fruit give you energy, while protein from lean meats, poultry, chicken, dairy products, soy, and legumes is required for growth and repair of tissues. Fat is needed for good health throughout your life span, especially in the first year of life, when it is necessary for proper brain development. Fat is a highly concentrated form of energy. Fat tastes good. It gives our food depth and richness. Our bodies crave it at times, and it helps bring on a feeling of

TRUTH

Banking calories lets you eat more on a special occasion.

If I know I'm going to a party on Saturday night and want the freedom to indulge a bit, here's what I do: I shave around 100 calories from what I normally eat Sunday through Friday and then have an extra 600 calories to play with by the time the party rolls around. Another option: Work out before the party. Walking four to six miles expends 400 to 600 calories.

fullness after eating a meal. The best strategy: Populate your plate with whole grains, vegetables, and fruits, modest helpings of protein, and a little fat.

HOW TO COUNT CALORIES WITHOUT REALLY COUNTING CALORIES

To successfully shed pounds, it's always good to keep track of calories. It's really easy to guess too low, however. Portion size can become so distorted, and we tend to think that our meals have fewer calories than they actually have. People who are overweight are especially likely to make this mistake, which may make it more difficult for them to lose weight.

Calories can be hidden everywhere—cappuccino with skim milk is fine, but whole milk adds an extra 20 to 30 calories. A large bagel is calorie dense and can run up to 400 calories. A lot of us just don't realize how calorie packed some foods are. Until you get familiar with the calorie counts of foods, try keeping a food journal in which you write down what you eat alongside each food's calorie count. When you write it down, you'll see exactly what, where, and when you're eating, which helps to identify—and change—your eating patterns. You may also find that you're spending more calories at one time of the day than another.

I would be lying to you if I said calorie counting was fun, however. Calculating calories every day is tedious busywork, unless you like that sort of thing. If not, try my "modular" approach. Simply package as much of your

TRUTH

There are no negative-calorie foods.

You may have heard that some foods, because they are difficult to digest, will make you lose weight. Dubbed "negative-calorie foods," citrus fruits and celery have both basked in this flattering light in fad diets over the years. The problem is that it's not true. The calories your body burns in fueling the digestive cycle are minuscule compared with the calories in the food itself. Although chewing celery might seem like a strenuous activity, it burns about the same amount of calories as watching grass grow.

food as possible into 100-calorie portions—100-calorie slices of lean proteins, servings of legumes, bags of cut-up veggies and fruit—or buy foods like yogurt that come in 100-calorie packages. Each day, instead of counting calories, you count food portions. Yes, it takes some prep time initially, but this method sure is easy. Once you do it for a while, you'll be able to eyeball your portions and know how many calories they have. See the chart on the next page for examples of 100-calorie portions of common foods. My Treat Yourself Diet (page 237) is put together in modular meals, with the day's calories already counted for you.

But watch out for "mini-packages." These are foods like cookies, candy, and snacks that come in small, premeasured 100-calorie-a-serving packages. While they offer a manageably sized treat, snack packs are still processed foods with sugar, salt, and saturated fats. Enjoying them once in a while won't hurt you or blow your diet, but if you snack on them every day or several times a day, the unhealthy effects are going to show up on your hips or tummy. And because some aren't very filling, you might be left craving even more food.

What You Get for 100 Calories

Breads, Cereals, and Grains
Bran flakes—¾ cup
Cornflakes—1 cup
Dinner roll, whole wheat—2½-inch diameter
Pancake, 4-inch diameter—1 cake
Pasta—½ cup cooked
Popcorn, oil popped—2 cups
Rice, long grained, white—½ cup cooked
Waffle—1 multigrain Belgian waffle

Dairy Foods
Cheese, full fat—1 ounce
Ice cream, no sugar added—½ cup
Low-fat milk, 1%—1 cup
Yogurt, light—6 ounces

Fruit
Applesauce, sweetened—½ cup
Avocado—½ of a small avocado
Banana—1 fruit
Mango, raw, sliced—1 cup
Orange—1 large 10-ounce fruit
Strawberries, raw—2 cups

Protein
Almonds or cashews—10 nuts
Egg—1 large
Fish, white—3 ounces
Hot dog, light—1 dog
Peanut butter—1 tablespoon
Roast beef, lean—2 ounces
Tuna, light, canned in water—3 ounces
Shrimp, boiled—3 ounces

Vegetables
Black beans—½ cup
Corn on the cob—1½ ears
Lettuce, shredded—10 cups
Peas—1 cup
Sweet potato, mashed—½ cup
Vegetables, mixed (broccoli, cauliflower, carrots)—3 cups cooked

Beverages
Distilled liquors, 80 proof—1 jigger
Lemonade, pink—1 cup
Light beer—1 can or bottle (12 fluid ounces)
Wine—5 ounces (full regular-sized wineglass)
Orange juice—1 cup

Another way to count calories without really counting them is to section off your plate. Fill one quarter of it with lean meat, chicken, or fish. This gives you the 3- to 4-ounce, 100-calorie serving recommended on most diets (it will be about the size of a deck of playing cards). Fill the next quarter of the plate with complex carbohydrates (beans, a baked sweet potato, or rice). This equals about a ½ cup serving, or around 100 calories. Finally, fill half your plate with nonstarchy vegetables (like broccoli, carrots, or lettuce). Proportioning your plate like this creates the right fuel mix and automatically slashes fat grams and calories to healthy levels.

The size of your plate makes a difference, too. Start using a salad plate as your dinner plate. This trick automatically cuts down your portion sizes. Europeans use smaller plates, and they don't have the weight problems Americans have. Just for kicks, line up a 9-inch plate, an 11-inch plate, and a 13-inch plate. You'll be shocked by the difference in their surface areas!

TRUTH

No-fat doesn't mean no-calorie.

These days, you can buy reduced-fat and fat-free versions of nearly all your favorite foods, from cookies to ice cream. The problem is, these foods still contain calories (usually from sugar) and the serving sizes can be deceptively small. So read labels carefully. Just because something is labeled "low fat" or "fat-free" doesn't mean you can eat all you want. Calories still count, even with diet foods.

For those of you who love those all-you-can-eat buffets, think twice. For a study that was published in 2008 in the journal *Obesity,* researchers at Cornell University dispatched observers to watch eating behaviors at these buffets. What they found was not surprising: the heaviest people used large plates; thinner people used smaller plates. Another tip that emerged from this study: Use chopsticks at a Chinese buffet instead of a fork. You'll eat less.

After you use any of these methods, even for a short time, you'll get to be a pro at calorie counting. Weight loss is a simple equation: calories in minus calories out. To knock off pounds, you have to understand this equation and be aware of your own numbers. You may feel that keeping tabs on them every day is a pain but if you don't, you won't lose weight. Your numbers don't lie.

TRUTH

As we get older our calorie needs go down and our protein needs go up.

This information is important. If you're maintaining your weight on 1,800 to 2,000 calories a day, you may want to bump that down by 100 to 200 calories daily by age sixty. One requirement that doesn't drop as we age, however, is our need for protein. The daily recommendation for protein is 46 grams for women and 56 grams for men. If you eat too little protein, your body may start drawing on muscle, and over time, any muscle loss can lead to weakness and lack of strength. Dietitians advise that older people should shoot for 1 gram of protein per kilogram of body weight. That equates roughly to half your weight in pounds. (So a 160-pound senior should try to eat 80 grams of protein a day.)

UNDERSTANDING LABEL CLAIMS

CLAIM	WHAT IT MEANS
Calorie-free	Less than 0.5 calorie per serving
Cholesterol-free	Fewer than 2 milligrams of cholesterol and 2 grams or fewer of saturated fat per serving
Fat-free	Less than 0.5 gram of fat per serving
Low fat	3 grams or fewer of total fat per serving
Low calorie	40 calories or fewer per serving
Low cholesterol	20 milligrams or fewer of cholesterol and 2 grams or fewer of saturated fat per serving
Low saturated fat	1 gram or less of saturated fat per serving and not more than 15 percent of calories from saturated fat
Low sodium	140 milligrams or fewer per serving
Very low sodium	35 milligrams or fewer per serving
Lean	Fewer than 10 grams of fat, 4.5 grams or fewer of saturated fat, and fewer than 95 milligrams of cholesterol per serving and per 100 grams
Extra lean	Fewer than 5 grams of fat, fewer than 2 grams of saturated fat, and fewer than 95 milligrams of cholesterol per serving and per 100 grams
Light or lite	One-third fewer calories; or no more than one-half the fat of the higher-calorie, higher-fat version; or no more than one-half the sodium of the higher-sodium version
Sugar-free	Less than 0.5 gram of sugar per serving

EXTRA, EXTRA

Don't Watch TV While Eating!

The average American watches about four hours of television a day, a habit that's been linked to obesity or being overweight in a number of studies. Watching television more than two hours a day also raises the risk of overweight in children, even in those as young as three years old. And studies show that eating food in front of the TV stimulates people to eat more calories—nearly 140 more calories per day, which adds up to an extra 14 pounds a year. If you must snack in front of the TV, try what my family does and munch on popcorn for a late-night snack.

Myth #4

Carbs Are Bad for You

I am married to a jock with a strong, fit body and a determined mind to match. By day, Doug is an Emmy Award–winning sports producer. After hours, he is passionate about exercise and many outdoor sports, including mountain biking, rowing, biking, and hiking. Committed to staying in shape, Doug knows his waist size and his muscle mass down to the exact measurements. He unconsciously touches his waist when he's had too much to eat and is intuitive about when he feels good and when he doesn't.

I remember a time a few years ago, during a particularly active summer, when Doug was downright exhausted after physical activity, and he couldn't understand why. He had just had a medical checkup and got a clean bill of health from his doctor.

I felt, however, that his diet was due for a checkup of

its own. At the time, Doug had fallen under the spell that says carbs are bad, so he was eating lots of protein and vegetables. Part of his regimen included protein shakes—it was rare for me to walk in the kitchen and not find a sticky blender. He loved those shakes. Occasionally, he would throw in some fruit, but not often, so he wasn't getting much of a carbohydrate bump from his shakes. Not only that, Doug hardly ever ate breakfast.

I suggested that he might be overtrained and under-nourished, which would be two simple reasons for his fatigue. When you're low on carbs, your body starts pulling energy from stored carbohydrate (glycogen). The dwindling down of those reserves will leave you feeling sluggish unless they're replaced by dietary carbs.

Doug was basically running on empty, and this was undercutting his energy. His body was crying out for carbs. Doug disagreed. Although he had basically pushed carbs off the table in favor of protein, he insisted that his diet was nutritious, so his lifestyle could not be blamed for his tiredness, he argued. Old habits die hard.

Let's at least put my theory to the test, I said, and at least Doug was receptive. We added more carbohydrates to his diet—whole-grain cereal at breakfast, a banana in his protein shakes, dark whole-grain bread for sandwiches, and brown rice or baked potatoes at dinner—all foods that in our carb-phobic society are considered bad for you.

Within days, Doug felt revived. He had given himself the proper resources to fuel his vigorous activities. He has told me more than once about how energized he feels by these tweaks to his diet. The lesson in this experience for him was: Carbs are not the enemy.

CARBS 101

Let's do a crash course on carbohydrates. What are carbs? Do they make us fat? How many do we really need? And how in the world should we keep track of them? It may seem complicated, but with a couple of tools, this is a slam dunk.

First, carbohydrates are, by definition, the sugars, starches, and fiber found in our food. The most common sugar is sucrose, which you know best as table sugar. Most plant foods, including cereals, whole grains, pasta, fruits, and vegetables, are starches, also called complex carbohydrates. Sugars and starches are our body's fuel of choice. The problem is, any excess fuel not burned is immediately stored in our fat cells. And once they set up camp, they are tough to kick out. Fiber is the indigestible remnant of plant food found in starches and in less starchy vegetables, and it keeps you regular.

TRUTH

You need carbs to burn fat.

Many dieters have forgotten that the body actually requires carbs to burn fat. As fat is broken down into energy, a series of complex chemical reactions takes place inside cells. Fat is like a log on a hearth waiting to be ignited. Carbohydrate is the match that ignites fat at the cellular level. Unless enough carbohydrate is available in key stages of the energy-producing process, fat will just smolder—in other words, not burn as cleanly or completely.

TRUTH

Carbs do not cause diabetes.

One of the more popularized beliefs is that you can give yourself type 2 diabetes by eating sugars or "bad carbs" because they cause blood sugar and insulin levels to surge. Not true. Diabetes is caused by a combination of genetic and lifestyle factors. Being overweight, however, does increase your risk for developing type 2 diabetes, so you do have to watch your calories from all foods, including carbs. If you have a history of diabetes in your family, you must take into account how to balance the foods you eat with the amount of exercise you get. Good nutrition and regular exercise are helpful tools in reducing the risk of this disease.

Carbs are also a primary source of vitamins, minerals, antioxidants, and phytochemicals. Foods with carbs include grains such as rice, wheat, barley, and oats; cereals, including packaged varieties; breads and pastas; beans and legumes; soy; all vegetables; all fruits; and sweets such as candy, soft drinks, jams and jellies, cakes, and any sugary food.

Carbs have been trashed, and we've been encouraged to refuse the bread basket, skip the white foods, and trade in potatoes for pork rinds. What gives? Why do we fear carbs so much, and why have they been so maligned? Blame it partially on the low-carb-diet craze of the past decade plus.

ANATOMY OF A MYTH

Low-carb diets have been with us for a long time. The first low-carb-diet guru, on the scene more than a century ago, was William Banting, who actually got his diet from his doctor, the British ear surgeon William Harvey. Banting had grown so fat in middle age that he could not climb upstairs for fear of being toppled by his own girth. Dr. Harvey prescribed a regimen focused on meat, small amounts of fruit, and liberal servings of wine and sherry, which helped Banting drop 35 pounds in thirty-eight weeks. Delighted by this result, Banting printed the diet at his own expense, called it *Banting's Letter on Corpulence,* and distributed thousands of free copies. The diet was so popular that when he died in 1878, nearly sixty thousand additional copies had been sold. Since Banting's background wasn't in health or medicine—he was an undertaker—this established the precedent that diet gurus need know nothing about nutrition or physiology.

It has been only in recent years, however, that the low-carb diet, typically defined as eating fewer than 90 grams daily of carbohydrates, has achieved such wide and sustained popularity. The most famous popularizer of low-carb diets was the American medical doctor Robert Atkins. Atkins suggested that when you reduce your carbohydrate consumption, the body's blood-sugar levels decrease and cause the pancreas to produce less insulin. With less insulin to draw on, the body is forced to burn fat reserves for energy, resulting in rapid weight loss. Eating more fat—a food category that formerly was taboo for many dieters—makes the body feel full, leading to fewer carbohydrate cravings. In addition to fats, other allowable foods are unlimited amounts of meats, cheeses, nonstarchy vegetables, and limited amounts of nuts and low-carb fruits such as strawberries and blueberries.

TRUTH

Nuts can be a part of a diet.

In small amounts, nuts have a place in a healthy weight-loss program. Nuts are high in calories and fat; there's no doubt about that. But many nuts contain healthy fats that do not clog arteries. Nuts are also good sources of protein, dietary fiber, and minerals, including magnesium and copper. Enjoy small portions of nuts, but keep in mind that one-half ounce of mixed nuts has about 270 calories. That's a small volume for a lot of fat, so choose wisely.

If you love nuts, those lowest in calories include pistachios, almonds, cashews, and peanuts (which are technically legumes) at around 160 calories per ounce.

Off-limits are honey, sugar in any form, breads, grains, and all starchy vegetables like potatoes. Thus, you can have a hamburger but no bun. Order eggs and bacon, but forget the toast. Feast on prime rib, butter, and sour cream, but ditch the baked potato. Do this faithfully, and you will lose weight. Many other low-carb diets were spawned, all with the same basic principle in common: Eat more protein and fewer carbohydrates and sugar.

Although hard to stick to, high-protein, low-carbohydrate diets do work for short-term weight loss, but it's because they greatly restrict your choices. Most Americans get more than half their calories from carbohydrates. Eat meals that reduce your carbohydrate access by half and you'll be hard pressed to make up the calories from fat and protein. In essence, then, you're restricting your calorie intake. That takes us back to the basic equation of weight loss: calories in and calories out.

As I explained in Myth #3, restricting calorie intake results in weight loss. When you look closely at studies in which people lost weight on low-carb diets, they generally ate fewer calories. The typical low-carb plan is around 1,400 calories per day. If you eat that way after eating 2,500 calories a day, the equation works in your favor. You're bound to knock off pounds.

On the flip side, there are still questions about the long-term health effects of a high-protein / low-carbohydrate diet. One thing scientists know is that much of the yummy stuff in low-carb diets—think prime rib and cheese—comes loaded with artery-clogging saturated fats. Low-carb mania has not upended the scientific consensus that saturated fats are the enemy—a major risk factor for heart disease and stroke.

I have never loved this approach to weight loss because getting most of your daily calories from high-protein foods like meat, eggs, and cheese is not balanced eating. If you're prone to constipation, low-carb diets can make matters worse as they tend to be low in fiber. They may also make you feel lethargic because the brain needs glucose to feel sharp. I have concerns that in the long run a very high intake of saturated fat and red meat is at odds with heart health and cancer prevention. There are at least four micronutrients—folate, potassium, vitamin C, and magnesium—that protect people from heart disease but can be deficient in low-carb dieters.

Because these diets are high in protein, they may burden the kidneys. Proteins contain nitrogen, which

TRUTH

Protein can make you fat.

Excess anything—protein, carbohydrates, or dietary fat—can make you pack on pounds. Let's say you require around 2,000 calories to maintain a healthy weight. And you meet that requirement, but enjoy a nice steak, even a protein shake, above those 2,000 calories. Trust me, the extra protein will be dispatched to the liver, converted to sugar, and eventually packed away as fat. Although protein is a little less efficient at manufacturing body fat than dietary fat and carbs are, don't be misled by diets that say you can eat all the protein you want and not gain weight.

the kidneys must remove from the body. So, the extra protein typical of low-carbohydrate diets makes the kidneys work harder than normal. This is a problem for people with diabetes who may already have kidney damage.

Low-carb dieting can lead to the buildup of ketones (partially broken-down fats) in your blood. Excessive ketones in your blood can poison the body; this is called ketosis. It can be especially risky for pregnant women and people with unchecked diabetes or kidney disease. Also, too much protein can leach calcium out of the body, increasing the risk of osteoporosis.

Finally, carbs in a meal induce insulin to trigger the delivery of tryptophan to the brain. That amino acid is involved in manufacturing the mood-enhancing brain neurotransmitter serotonin. Without enough carbs to complete this transaction, you could end up feeling moody, depressed, and low on energy.

TRUTH

Fiber fights fat.

How much fiber we eat affects our risk for obesity. It wasn't always that way, but these days people are eating half the fiber required by the body for good health (remember, we need between 25 and 35 grams a day). Fiber makes you feel full, stimulates the release of appetite-suppressing hormones in the gut, naturally binds to fat and escorts it out of the body, and helps regulate blood sugar. Include more high-fiber foods in your diet, like legumes, whole grains, fruits, and vegetables, and you'll go a long way toward keeping your weight in check. This is an incredibly easy, no-willpower way to manage your weight with good carbs.

But the low-carb diet craze is not the only reason carbs are seen as bad guys: When they hang out with the wrong crowd, like processing machines that strip away their fiber, vitamins, and minerals, carbs do go bad. Think healthy potato turned fattening potato chip. Also, many carbs, like bread, rice, pasta, cereal, beans, fruits, and some vegetables (like potatoes and yams), become high in fat and calories when eaten in large portion sizes or when covered with high-fat toppings like butter, sour cream, or mayonnaise.

DO CARBS MAKE YOU FAT?

Carbohydrates can contain a lot of calories, but oddly, that's not the main reason they're shunned for weight loss. It's more for their effect on insulin, the hormone that helps your body assimilate sugar (glucose) and turns the sugar into energy. When you eat a lot of processed carbs (think junk food), the level of glucose in your bloodstream spikes. Insulin, produced by your pancreas, is released to lower it. Insulin is also a fat storage hormone; it helps convert excess glucose in the bloodstream into fat.

The problem isn't carbs, since carbohydrates per se do not make us fat. What we're doing wrong that allows for so many Americans to be either overweight or obese is eating too many calories from carbs and other foods. If you're not burning off those calories, you'll likely store more fat.

By contrast, look at the French. They are known for their rich, Continental cuisine, yet obesity is relatively rare in France. Many years ago I was lucky enough to have dinner in Paris with the iconic cook Julia Child, who specialized in French cooking. Anyone who is familiar with Julia knows that she loved food with a passion—and that means the real thing, not the low-calorie substitutes that so many Americans are devouring. So we had wine, which she fervently believed is good for the palate, the digestion, and yes, the heart. The four people at our table ordered a variety of foods—all rich in carbohydrates and fat. But here was the catch: Julia ate only enough to satisfy her desire for the food. Never fooled by the notion of needing to finish everything, she didn't clean her plate. She tasted and enjoyed—in very small portions. Julia believed that food was for taste, and for the conviviality of those gathered to enjoy it.

In France, the croissants, glasses of wine, even portions served at McDonald's, are smaller than ours. When

TRUTH

By itself, fiber may not be enough to protect you from colon cancer.

Colon cancer killed my grandfather, and my father overcame it twenty-five years ago, so this is a subject I have followed carefully. Fiber turns out to be only one part of the protection picture. With two generations affected in my family, I know I am at risk, so I watch what I eat and get a colonoscopy each year. But prevention goes even further. Studies suggest a possible correlation between cigarette smoking and cancer of the colon—another reason to quit, if you haven't already.

Here's my advice: Though we don't have all the answers yet, stick with the fiber because it's good for you. It lowers cholesterol levels and protects against high blood pressure and heart disease. And it is also good for your gut, even if it doesn't turn out to be a colon-cancer preventer. Then, look carefully at your lifestyle and your family tree. If you have any questions about your risk or what tests you should be getting, talk with your doctor.

the French and other Europeans come to the United States, they are stunned by the size of our plates and portions. We are literally expanding our waistlines with our portions and the glut of calories taken in as a result. It's so easy to add 200 calories here and 300 there. And before you know it, you have another pound or two staring back at you from the scale.

It's also picking the right carbs that matters to your health. For instance, it's better to choose brown rice over white because it contains more fiber (which will fill you up) and more than three times the amount of vitamin E. So forget the crazy myth that *all* carbs are bad for you. Not true! Natural and minimally processed carbs like the ones listed next are important to your health. Here are your best carbohydrate bets:

Whole grains and whole wheat pasta. Foods like oatmeal, rice, barley, and whole wheat products are not fattening and are loaded with nutrients and fiber. They also taste great. On the whole, they are low in fat and calories and are filling. They keep you full so you don't overeat and put on pounds. There is strong scientific evidence that people who have a higher intake of whole grains, or who increase their intake of whole grains, gained less weight than those who have a very low intake of whole grains. That's plausible because whole grains make people feel full. Eating more whole grains has also been shown to pare down belly fat.

TRUTH

Broccoli and blueberries are "perfect" foods.

Few foods measure up to broccoli and blueberries for their disease-fighting potential. Broccoli is rich in sulforaphane, an antioxidant linked with a reduced risk of a number of cancers, especially lung, stomach, colon, and rectal cancers. Broccoli also has anti-inflammatory properties, and we know that an important factor in reducing the risk of disease is to decrease inflammation. Blueberries are rich in anthocyanidins, compounds that help protect the heart and may inhibit the growth of cancer cells. Studies suggest the blueberry anthocyanidins protect against neurodegenerative diseases like Alzheimer's and Parkinson's and can slow and even reverse age-related memory loss. It's not clear how much of these foods you need to eat, but it makes sense to include more broccoli and blueberries in your diet.

High-fiber cereals. We need 25 to 35 grams of fiber daily, and high-fiber cereals are an easy way to get it. Read labels and look for cereals that contain more than 3 grams of fiber per serving; this amount qualifies it as a high-fiber food. Natural grain cereals like oatmeal and Cream of Wheat are great, too.

Bread, bread, and more bread. I think bread is one of the greatest gifts on earth. It has been used by various civilizations for centuries and should be consumed with great joy. It is the cornerstone of diets all over the world

TRUTH

White foods can be good for your health.

Some diets admonish: "Eat nothing white!" This advice comes from the idea that some highly processed foods, especially those made with lots of sugar and white flour, are not good for you—and can make you fat. Many white foods, however, are very healthy. Cauliflower is white, yet full of vitamins and phytochemicals—not to mention, it's low in calories. Other healthful white foods are potatoes, white beans, onions, garlic, and soy foods like tofu. As for potatoes, lots of nutrients are in the skin, so eat the whole potato.

Postscript: I used to eat white rice and brown rice. Then I learned that there are some big nutritional differences between the two. White rice is far less nutritious than brown rice. By comparison, a cup of cooked brown rice has 4.8 grams of fiber, while white rice has almost none. White rice is also higher in calories: 120 calories in a half-cup serving. To make up for its shortcomings, white rice is often enriched with iron and other nutrients. Even so, white rice is one "white food" I no longer buy.

where obesity is rarely encountered. Good bread is not fattening. It's what we put on it that does us in. Eat bread and enjoy it. Reach for whole-grain varieties with at least 2 grams of fiber per slice. Whole wheat and high-fiber pitas and tortillas are terrific, too.

Fruits and vegetables. You just can't go wrong with this group of carbs. Fruits and vegetables are loaded with vitamins, minerals, antioxidants, and a variety of natural plant chemicals called phytochemicals that have wide-ranging health benefits. Foods that are rich in vitamin C may offer protection from cancer and help absorb iron from foods. These include broccoli, peppers, citrus fruits,

TRUTH

Frozen and canned fruits and veggies can be just as nutritious as fresh.

Frozen or canned produce is often packaged right after it has been picked, which helps keep most of its nutrients. Fresh produce can sometimes lose nutrients after being exposed to light or air. I had a habit of buying lots of fresh vegetables but not eating them before they spoiled. Now I cook them before they ever get to the fridge. Some canned produce can be more nutritious than fresh, since certain antioxidants like the lycopene in tomatoes and beta-carotene in carrots are more easily absorbed in the body if the vegetable has been cooked. The recommended intake of fruits and vegetables for adults is 7 to 13 servings per day. Incorporating fresh as well as frozen increases your chances of getting all those servings in.

strawberries, kiwi, cantaloupes, and tomatoes. Eating a vegetable-and-fruit-based diet helps you get the greatest variety of nutrients. An easy way to make this a habit is to simply eat one or more servings a day from each of these categories of fruits and vegetables:

Citrus fruits

Noncitrus fruits, including berries

Green and dark green leafy vegetables, including spinach and romaine lettuce

Yellow/orange or red vegetables such as sweet peppers, carrots, squash, and sweet potatoes. The more colorful the fruit or vegetable, the higher it is in nutrients and disease-fighting antioxidants.

Cruciferous vegetables like broccoli, brussels sprouts, and cabbage, which contain cancer-fighting phyto-chemicals. (The reproductive structures of these foods contain components that are arranged like a cross, hence the name cruciferous, which derives from a word meaning "to place on a cross or crucify.")

Peas and legumes. These energy-loaded foods include black beans, black-eyed peas, chickpeas (garbanzo beans), kidney beans, soybeans and soy foods, and split peas. These carbs are also high in protein—the reason they're often staples in vegetarian diets. They're also extremely high in fiber and are packed with vitamins, especially B vitamins; and minerals like calcium, iron, potassium, magnesium, and zinc. If you're going to be a vegetarian, beans can be a mainstay of your diet.

Dairy products. We normally think of dairy products as a protein, which they are, but they do hold an appreciable amount of carbohydrate—in the form of lactose. Lactose is important because it stimulates the absorption of calcium from your intestine. One of the real concerns about including dairy in the diet is that some of it tends to be high in fat. There are really no hard-and-fast rules about what type of dairy to eat. But here are the guidelines I use: Limit hard cheeses because they're high in fat and enjoy them as a treat. Choose low-fat alternatives, such as low-fat milk and low-fat yogurt.

As for whole milk, most adults don't need it. As scientific investigators have traced the causes of heart disease, cancer, arthritis, migraines, and digestive problems, one suspect keeps coming up again and again: milk. Studies now link the epidemics of prostate cancer, digestive problems, and other ills to our habitual consumption of specific foods including—and especially—milk.

But doesn't drinking milk help strengthen bones and protect against osteoporosis? The Harvard Nurses' Health Study followed women for eighteen years, finding that milk drinkers had no protection against fractures, compared with women who drank little or no milk. Another study found that vegetarian women at age eighty had bones as dense as nonvegetarians at age sixty. This twenty-year advantage may have resulted from the lower protein intake of vegetarians. A high-protein diet increases the excretion of calcium.

We can get bone-strengthening calcium from plant sources such as beans, greens, whole-grain bread, tortillas, fortified juices, cereals, and nondairy milk. Nondairy milk includes soy milk, rice milk, and almond milk. Ounce for ounce, soy milk contains about the same amount of protein found in cow's milk, but the advantage of soy is that its protein comes from a purely vegetable source. Vegetable proteins are known to generate less calcium loss through the kidneys. All in all, nondairy milk alternatives are a great way to cut back on animal products, enjoy numerous health benefits, and satisfy your palate at the same time.

TRUTH

Bananas are a great diet food.

I confess that bananas are not my favorite food. I'm a picky banana eater; the fruit can't be too green or too ripe. But aside from my personal preferences, bananas have certainly gotten a bad rap, to the point of being banished from a lot of popular diets. Their exile comes from the glycemic index (GI), a tool that rates carbohydrates based on the speed at which they digest. GI proponents say that bananas are low in fiber but high in sugar, so they should be avoided. Nonsense. First off, bananas are low in calories (each one has about 100 calories) and low in fat. Plus, they contain "resistant starch," a component of some carbs that bypasses digestion—so a portion of the calories passes right through your body. Bananas bring many trace elements and antioxidants to your diet. They also contain 25 percent of the recommended minimum daily amount of potassium for adults. This makes them ideal for people who work out and lose potassium in sweat, or for elderly people who lose potassium from diuretics. Bananas are far richer in this important element than many other fruits.

HOW MANY CARBS DO YOU REALLY NEED?

One way to figure your daily carb allotment is this: Get 45 to 65 percent of your daily calories from carbohydrates. This calculation really isn't tricky. Decide how many calories you need to eat in a day to lose weight. For most sensible dieters, 1,200 calories a day should do it for women, and 1,500 to 1,800 calories for men. Multiply that number by .45, if you're using the 45 percent recommendation. Then divide that number by 4, since there are 4 calories in a gram of carbohydrate. That will give you the total number of carbohydrate grams you should eat in one day.

So it works like this:

1,200 calories × 0.45 = 540
540/4 = 135 grams of carbohydrate

Incidentally, adults require a *minimum* of 130 grams of carbohydrates a day, according to the "daily reference intake," a way of rating what we need for good health. Translating this into everyday foods, this is the same as: 8 slices of whole-grain bread or 3 cups of bran flakes or 6 medium apples or 3 medium baked potatoes. There are small paperback books that can give you the calorie, carbohydrate, and fat content of most foods; and the nutritional labeling on commercially prepared foods makes the task simple. As long as you eat in a balanced way—with plenty of vegetables and fruits—you'll obtain what you need without having to fuss with counting.

Natural carbohydrates are always the best, especially

TRUTH

You can eat after 8 P.M. and not gain weight.

It doesn't matter what time of day you eat. It is what and how much you eat and how much physical activity you do during the whole day that determines whether you gain, lose, or maintain your weight. No matter when you eat, your body will store extra calories as fat. If you want a snack before bedtime, think first about how many calories you've eaten that day.

fruits, vegetables, whole grains, and beans. It is the sugary and starchy man-made carbohydrates like candy bars, cakes, cookies, white bread, white rice, and chips that will do us in.

WHO SHOULD GO HIGH, WHO SHOULD GO LOW?

It's okay to use 130 grams as a baseline, but aim higher if you're exercising most days of the week. Serious exercisers and athletes like my husband need more carbs (at least 65 to 75 percent of your total daily calories, say sports nutritionists). The primary fuel for all body movement is glucose. With exercise, stores of carbohydrates (glycogen) in muscles and the liver are used rapidly, and carbohydrates are necessary to maintain the level of these body stores of readily utilizable fuel. Too much loss of glycogen from muscles is a big problem because this depletion will reduce physical performance and can cause premature fatigue. Carbs are a must-have when you're trying to develop body-toning muscle tissue. They fuel your body for exercise and help drive protein into muscles for growth.

TRUTH

A low-cal shake curbs the appetite.

Shakes are often pumped full of air, which tricks your stomach into thinking it's full so you eat less at each meal. Just make sure it's a low-cal shake such as some soy milk blended with fruit and crushed ice—or else you're defeating the purpose.

Some people will tell you they have trouble processing carbohydrates. This condition is related to "insulin resistance." Insulin, acting like the doorman of the bloodstream, instructs glucose in the blood to enter cells, where it is stored or used for energy. With insulin resistance, cells resist insulin's commands. What triggers insulin resistance? That's the great mystery, but many researchers think there is a genetic component, made worse by being overweight or inactive. When cells don't respond, more and more insulin is needed to do its job. The pancreas pumps out greater amounts of insulin until the hormone finally overwhelms the cells' resistance and forces glucose in. When the pancreas can no longer keep up with the need for more insulin, blood glucose levels stay constantly elevated. This condition, which is a problem of blood chemistry, can be the prelude to type 2 diabetes. Experts estimate that sixty million to seventy-five million Americans are insulin resistant, which is to say, teetering on the precipice of developing diabetes.

Many people who are insulin resistant, however, do not develop diabetes, because they are ultimately able to produce enough insulin to keep blood sugar from rising too high. However, excess insulin in the blood is not good. It can cause metabolic syndrome, a cluster of metabolic problems that raise the risk of heart disease.

If your doctor suspects you are insulin resistant, keeping your blood sugar under control is of primary importance, and your diet becomes a big deal. I would go far enough to say that your diet becomes your second job. Most researchers recommend a diet of at least 40 percent to 45 percent carbohydrates (remember the complex carbs such as beans, sweet potatoes, and brown rice, since simple carbs are metabolized directly into glucose), 35 percent to 40 percent fats (with an emphasis on foods rich in monounsaturated fats, like olive and canola oils and nuts, which help keep insulin and "bad" low-density lipoproteins in control), and 15 percent to 20 percent of calories from protein. This mix of macronutrients limits the strain on insulin production.

Even though we debate ad nauseam about carbs, and it gets confusing, I don't think nutrition is all that hard to figure out. Cut down on nutritionally bankrupt foods like sugar, junk food, and alcohol. Make sure you don't overindulge in fat. Get enough protein, and eat more vegetables, fruits, and whole grains. My mother has a great philosophy when looking at tempting food: "Is it worth wasting the calories?" she asks herself. Sometimes the answer is yes; sometimes it's no. One of the many things I learned from my mother is that life is all about balance and that the race is to the moderate.

What's the bottom line, then? Carbohydrates make life fun. They are good. They are not inherently unhealthy. Carbohydrates are a necessary friend and help round out a balanced diet. Make peace with them and move on.

EXTRA, EXTRA

Risk for diabetes and heart disease reversed in three weeks!

Can you lower risk for type 2 diabetes and cardiovascular disease in just three short weeks? Researchers from UCLA say yes. In the online *Journal of Applied Physiology,* they reported on a study testing the impact of a three-week diet combined with daily exercise among male participants ages forty-six to seventy-six. The team found that a nutrient-dense, high-fiber, low-fat diet together with daily aerobic exercise (forty-five to sixty minutes) effectively reversed metabolic syndrome and type 2 diabetes among study participants. Additionally, the program improved factors that contribute to heart disease, including insulin resistance, high cholesterol, oxidative stress, inflammation, and markers of atherosclerosis development—all achieved in less than one month.

Myth #5

Carbs Are Good for You

My brother and his wife thought their fifteen-year-old son Bryan was dying. For several years, he suffered digestive problems, mostly chronic diarrhea and abdominal pain. He lost so much weight that people thought he was anorexic. His hair was falling out. He was plagued with severe fatigue that did not go away, even when he got adequate rest.

Several doctors tried but failed to make sense of Bryan's symptoms. They diagnosed ulcers, colitis, migraines, chronic fatigue syndrome—and treatments to boot. Nothing worked. He underwent an endoscopy. But since he was a growing teenager, doctors were having trouble zeroing in on the problem.

Desperate but not willing to give up, Bryan's parents sent him to a specialist for allergy testing. They had already noticed that Bryan's symptoms would flare up the instant he ate certain foods like bread and pasta. Within days, the family had obtained a formal diagnosis: Bryan had celiac disease, an inherited immune disorder, and it would sentence him for life to not eating anything that contains wheat gluten or similar proteins in barley and rye. In his small intestine, those grain components triggered a chain of events causing bloating, diarrhea, and eventually malnutrition. No matter how much this growing teen ate, his body was, in effect, starving. Celiac disease can lead to fatigue, migraines, dermatitis, anemia, osteoporosis, even intestinal cancer.

Gluten is a complex protein and the second most prevalent food substance in Western civilization after sugar. In someone with celiac sprue, normal digestion doesn't completely break it down. Surviving pieces called peptides come in contact with the lining of the small intestine and the molecules of the immune system there. This molecular encounter results in an immune overreaction. Under the skirmish, that stretch of the digestive tract becomes inflamed and loses its villi, which are tiny, finger-like projections that normally provide a vast surface area for absorbing digested nutrients. The bowel recognizes the proteins as foreign invaders—a situation that causes the cramping, diarrhea, and many of the symptoms of celiac disease.

The only cure for celiac disease is a gluten-free diet. People who are diagnosed with the disease must give up not only most grain-based foods but also soups, sauces, canned foods, and hundreds of other items. This is because manufacturers frequently add gluten to processed foods, and they charge a hefty price for gluten-free products prepared instead with rice proteins and other alternative ingredients. But once you modify your diet, the symptoms will disappear. Going gluten-free usually heals the intestinal lining in about six months, but the diet must be followed for as long as you live.

Not many kids can imagine a world without cereal, pizza, or cookies. But these are just a few of the foods that Bryan's parents had to teach their son to avoid. Bryan isn't alone in enduring his gluten-free lifestyle.

Although celiac disease was considered rare in the United States a decade ago, recent tallies indicate that as many as one in every one hundred to two hundred people in the United States suffers from it. The diagnosis can be made via a simple antibody blood test; however, celiac disease is easily missed because the symptoms so closely mimic those of other conditions, such as lactose intolerance and irritable bowel syndrome. Many people with the condition aren't properly diagnosed and suffer its unexplained symptoms and potentially grave complications.

With his parents' help, Bryan began to adjust his diet. No more bread, cake, or cookies. And no more pizza, pasta, pretzels, fried chicken, crackers, or breakfast cereals—at least not the common versions of those foods. No more of anything that contained even a little wheat, rye, or barley.

As a newly diagnosed teen, it wasn't cool for Bryan to even ask what was in food he ordered and certainly not fun to not eat pizza at the local pizza parlor with his friends or turn down birthday cake at a birthday party. But eventually, being able to stave off the horrible symptoms and feel healthy again was worth signing on for, and Bryan became an experienced label reader, scanning the ingredient lists for sneaky gluten-containing ingredients such as farina, flour, caramel coloring, enriched flour, cereal, malt flavoring or extracts, MSG, modified food starch, semolina, and others.

Eventually, Bryan started living like any other kid but with restrictions. Before his diagnosis, he saw himself as a sick kid. But within a year, his life turned around, and his body felt strong again. And now, luckily, celiac-friendly, gluten-free foods are easy to find at most grocery stores.

In Bryan's case—and in the lives of the two million Americans with celiac disease—certain carbs are not good. They're not just bad; they can be life threatening. For them, "carbs are good" is definitely a myth.

But what about the rest of us? Is it accurate to lump all carbs in the same bread basket? Or are all carbs "good"? Are there "bad carbs"? If so, what are they?

The truth is that there are good carbs and bad carbs, just as there are good fats and bad fats. The so-called bad carbs are foods with lots of added sugar (sodas and candy) and refined starches (white bread, cookies, pastries, many crackers and cereals, and other white-flour products). They get their reputation because they are calorie rich and nutrient poor and provide little long-term satisfaction. So you eat more to get full, adding on pounds in the process. The "good carbs" I talked about in the previous chapter—whole fiber-filled starches (whole wheat pasta, vegetables, beans) are digested more slowly, so they fill you up, and they keep your blood sugar and insulin levels on an even keel.

TRUTH

Low carb doesn't necessarily mean low cal.

Today, food makers everywhere hawk low-carbohydrate products, including low-carb beer, bread, ice cream, and yes, even potatoes. Yet some low-carb products are so loaded with extra calories that they pose an unnecessary hurdle to weight loss. Take Subway's traditional 280-calorie 6-inch sandwich, for example. That's about half the calories of the low-carb Subway chicken bacon ranch wrap. Companies are reducing carb counts by replacing sugar and wheat flour with artificial sweeteners, sugar alcohols, and soy flour. But that doesn't mean you can eat low-carb ice cream with abandon. Scarfing down low-carb burgers, low-carb shakes, and low-carb fries will ultimately pack on unwanted pounds.

ANATOMY OF A MYTH

I believe that the dual myths of good carbs and bad carbs have been fueled not only by diet books that promote low-carb eating as the panacea for being overweight but also by a tool known as the glycemic index (GI) of foods, which assigns each food a numerical value based on how quickly it increases a person's blood glucose. Bad carbs are said to rate high on the GI. High-index carbs include sugars and easily digested starches; healthier carbs are lower on the index and include those found in whole grains, brown rice, fruits, and vegetables. These produce slower rises in blood sugar and a more tempered release of insulin, the hormone involved in moving glucose out of the bloodstream and into the cells, where it is used as fuel or stored as fat.

TRUTH

Mixed meals keep you satisfied.

It bears repeating that high-fiber, low-fat foods—whole grains, vegetables, fruits—should be the mainstay of your diet. Just be sure to eat them in combination with moderate helpings of protein. While carbs fill you up initially, they leave the stomach faster than protein. Protein with a little fat helps slow that process. So to stay satisfied for as long as possible, include a well-rounded mix at each meal. Aim to get 45 to 65 percent of calories from complex carbs (pasta, whole grain, breads), 15 to 20 percent from protein (lean cuts of beef, skinless chicken), and no more than 20 to 30 percent from fat.

Originally developed as a tool to keep diabetics' blood sugar even, a diet consisting of low-glycemic foods also seems to lower a healthy person's risk of developing diabetes and heart disease, probably because it limits the damage that elevated blood sugar inflicts on cells. Some experts think a low-glycemic diet also helps people lose weight, because smoothing out fluctuations in blood sugar may curb appetite—and there is credible scientific research to back this up.

Despite the possible health benefits of a low-glycemic diet, I'm not one for obsessing over the values that the index assigns to specific foods. Use common sense as a guide. For me, keeping track of GI issues is too laborious, and sometimes doesn't make sense. Potato chips, for example, score lower on the GI than air-popped popcorn, yet chips contain unhealthy amounts of saturated fat that aren't in unbuttered popcorn.

TRUTH

You don't have to eat low-glycemic carbs to lose weight.

The GI rates carbs based on the speed at which they digest. In theory, faster-digesting carbs are more efficient at stimulating the fat-storing process, and thus should be avoided if you're watching your waistline. Combining high-protein foods with fast-digesting carbs or fiber-rich vegetables such as broccoli, cauliflower, spinach, mushrooms, and green beans will skew the index rating. For example, rice cakes, which are digested very fast, digest markedly slower when combined with sliced turkey, fat-free cheese or peanut butter, and even more slowly if you add in a small portion of vegetables as well. Combinations like this change the index rating—and benefit you and your waist.

The quality of the carbs you eat is what counts in weight management. The healthiest diet is also one of the simplest—loaded with fruits, vegetables, and whole grains—a diet that turns out to be low on the GI anyway.

THE SCOOP ON SUGAR

If there's a villain in the midst of carbs, I'd say it's mostly added sugars—the various types of sweeteners dumped into foods by manufacturers (and sometimes by us, when we spoon out table sugar). The USDA Dietary Guidelines has identified sugar as a part of our diet that we should limit. Why? Consuming lots of high-sugar foods, such as cookies and soft drinks, can lead not only to weight gain but also to nutrient deficiencies, since sugary foods often replace more nutritious fare. It's not a reach to say that people who eat larger amounts of sugar generally have the worst diets. Data from a national nutrition survey revealed that as sugar increases in the diet, intakes of calcium, vitamin A, iron, and zinc decrease.

Sucrose, or table sugar, is added to many packaged and processed foods, including desserts and snacks. Likewise, high-fructose corn syrup, a chemically altered form of the natural sugar fructose, is added to soft drinks, many fruit drinks, and sweets that have little or no redeeming nutritional value. Once in the body, high-fructose corn syrup raises total cholesterol levels, low-density lipoproteins (harmful LDL cholesterol), and triglycerides.

Fructose is also bad for your waistline. In research, overweight adults who consumed large amounts of fructose experienced alarming changes in body fat and insulin sensitivity (meaning insulin had a harder time doing its job). These changes do not occur after eating glucose. In a study conducted at the University of California–Davis, those given fructose saw an increase in abdominal fat, the kind that wraps around your internal organs, causes a potbelly, and has been linked to an increased risk of diabetes and cardiovascular disease. This did not happen with the group who consumed glucose, even though both groups gained around 4 pounds in weight. Because this study looked only at pure fructose, not high-fructose corn syrup or sucrose, it is not yet clear whether these substances are to blame for the epidemic of obesity and diabetes, but I have my suspicion that they contribute. If you want to keep your waistline nice and trim, it's probably not a good idea to eat too much high-fructose corn syrup.

TRUTH

Juices can expand your waistline.

Sure, fruit juice is a better choice than soda. Juice is convenient and tastes great, but it doesn't have the fiber of the original fruit. And many juice drinks may contain more water and sugar than actual fruit. Most of us drink more juice than we realize. A true serving is no more than a half cup. A large glass can contain twice that amount. (Check your mother's or grandmother's cupboard for an old juice glass; you'll be shocked by its tiny size.) Because fruit juice packs a lot of calories in a small space, if you're watching your weight, it's smarter to grab a piece of fruit.

Fruit contains a lot of naturally occurring sugar as fructose, which most low-carb diets also limit or shun completely. But unless you have a metabolic problem

TRUTH

"Net carbs" is an unscientific term.

Food manufacturers claim that because fiber isn't digested and sugar alcohols have a negligible effect on blood glucose, and therefore a minimal effect on weight gain, they do not count. It's true that fiber passes through the digestive system largely intact and sugar alcohols have a minimal impact on blood glucose. But here's where the math gets fuzzy: Sugar alcohols have a significant amount of calories and thus *do* count. Every gram of sugar—refined, unrefined, or sugar alcohol—is 4 calories. Your weight is affected by the amount of calories you eat and the amount of energy you expend. Read labels and compare the calories in low-carb versus regular foods. They're often either close or the same.

that prevents you from digesting fructose, few experts suggest cutting back your intake of fruit, except perhaps if you get your fruit from juice, because it's so concentrated and packs in a lot of calories and sugar. You'd do better to eat more fresh fruit and less juice anyway, especially since fruit contains more fiber. Fruit, despite consisting almost entirely of carbs, is also an excellent source of vitamins, minerals, and phytochemicals.

HOW MUCH SUGAR IS TOO MUCH?

Should sugar be a forbidden fruit, so to speak? Not exactly. The occasional dessert after a healthful meal is just fine. So is the occasional piece of candy. I periodically munch on a couple of Gummi Bears at work to satisfy my sweet tooth. It's when sodas, cakes, cookies, and doughnuts become menu mainstays that your diet—and possibly your health—is in trouble. There are many health concerns about sugar, including its possible role in diseases like obesity, diabetes, hyperactivity, and tooth decay. The only proven link, however, is between sugar and tooth decay. A diet high in sugar or carbs doesn't cause diabetes, as I mentioned earlier, but it may make you overweight, which is a risk factor for type 2 diabetes. Cutting back on your intake to lose weight may decrease your chance of getting diabetes.

Nor is there any scientific evidence that sugar triggers hyperactivity in children. But it will make them obese. Further, many high-sugar foods are loaded with fat—so if your kids are eating a lot of sugar- and fat-laced foods, they'll start putting on pounds, even to the point of being

TRUTH

Raisins fight tooth decay.

Medical experts used to think that sweet, sticky foods (like raisins) caused tooth decay. But scientists have now found that raisins fight bacteria in the mouth that cause cavities and gum disease. A study conducted by University of Illinois researchers showed that several chemicals in this popular snack food suppress the growth of several species of oral bacteria associated with cavities and gum disease. So consider raisins a healthy food, but don't go overboard. One cup of raisins packs around 493 calories.

at greater risk for "adult" diseases like type 2 diabetes and heart disease. The goal isn't to eliminate sugar from your diet but to include it in appropriate amounts.

What do I mean by "appropriate"? Here, experts differ. The World Health Organization advocates limiting intake of sugars to below 10 percent of your daily calories. If you eat 1,800 calories a day, that translates into 180 calories a day from sugar, or about 12 teaspoons. If that sounds like a lot, it is. But most Americans eat twice that amount of sugar, if not more, every day.

To give you an idea of how far that daily sugar quota might go, a piece of cake with icing has about 4 teaspoons of sugar, one milk chocolate bar has around 5 teaspoons of sugar, and a soft drink packs 10 teaspoons. You can figure out the teaspoons of sugar yourself. Check the Nutrition Facts label. "Total sugar" is listed on the Nutrition Facts label in grams. If you divide the number of grams by 4, you'll get the approximate number of teaspoons of sugar in the food. This tally does not account for natural sugar, but if sugar is one of the first ingredients on the label, most of the sugar is probably added.

Sugar is lurking everywhere—in places where you would least expect it. And many food manufacturers don't make it easy on us because they list the sugar in foods by many different names (see the chart below), so you've got to be a savvy label reader.

A SUGAR BY ANY OTHER NAME . . .

The best way to know whether added sugars are a major ingredient is to read the ingredient list. Look for the terms listed below, and remember, the closer they are to the beginning of the ingredient list, the bigger the percentage of sugar in the product.

Barley malt	A sweetener produced from sprouted barley that is mostly maltose. It is used in combination with other sweeteners and for cooking and baking.
Brown rice syrup	A sweetener produced commercially by cooking brown rice flour or brown rice starch with enzymes. It can be used for cooking and baking and is sometimes combined with fruit concentrates to be used in food products.
Brown sugar	A refined sugar coated with molasses.
Cane syrup	A very sweet syrup made from sugarcane.
Corn syrup	A manufactured syrup of cornstarch that contains varying proportions of glucose, maltose, and dextrose. It is used in salad dressings, tomato sauces, powdered drink mixes, fruit drinks and juices, and desserts like pudding and ice milk.
Crystalline fructose	A sweetener that is made from cornstarch and comes in granules like table sugar. It is used in dry mix beverages, low-calorie products, enhanced or flavored water, still and carbonated beverages, sports and energy drinks, chocolate milk, breakfast cereals, baked goods, yogurt, fruit packs, and confections.

A SUGAR BY ANY OTHER NAME . . .

Dextrose	Another name for glucose. A simple sugar that is less sweet than fructose or sucrose. It is used in many baking products like cake mixes and frostings, snack foods like cookies, crackers, and pretzels, and desserts like custards and sherbets.
Fructose	A sugar found naturally in fruit; also a simple sugar refined from fruit.
High fructose corn syrup	A highly concentrated syrup of mostly fructose and some glucose that is prevalent in soft drinks and other processed foods.
Honey	A concentrated solution of fructose and glucose, plus some sucrose. It is produced by bees from the nectar of flowers.
Invert sugar	A sugar created by heating sugar syrup with a small amount of acid such as cream of tartar or lemon juice in order to reduce the size of the sugar crystals. The resulting product is smoother and suitable for use in candies and some syrups.
Lactose	A simple sugar in milk.
Maltodextrin	A sugar made from maltose and dextrose in corn. It is used in a wide array of foods, from canned fruits to snacks.
Maltose	A simple sugar made from starch.
Mannitol, sorbitol, xylitol	Sugar alcohols derived from fruit or produced from dextrose. These sweeteners are used in many dietetic products. Sugar alcohols do not promote tooth decay, unlike sugar.
Maple syrup	A concentrated sap from maple trees, predominantly fructose.
Molasses	The thick syrup by-product from the processing of sugarcane or sugar beet into sugar. Blackstrap molasses, a popular health food, is a good source of calcium, iron, and potassium.
Muscovado or Barbados sugar	A British specialty brown sugar that is very dark brown and has a particularly strong molasses flavor. The crystals are slightly coarser and stickier in texture than "regular" brown sugar.
Sucanat	Nonrefined cane sugar that retains all of its molasses content.

A SUGAR BY ANY OTHER NAME . . .

Sucrose	Refined, crystallized sap of the sugarcane or sugar beet; a combination of glucose and fructose.
Turbinado	A less refined sugar that still has some natural molasses coating.
White grape juice	A highly purified fructose solution. Virtually no other nutrients are present. It is often used in juice concentrate blends.

TRUTH

Cookie dough can harbor salmonella.

If you love baking holiday cookies with your kids, be careful about licking the bowl. The salmonella bacterium—which causes an infection marked by vomiting and diarrhea—has been linked to uncooked eggs, which unfortunately are in cookie dough. I've had this infection, and I felt so miserable I thought I was going to die. The good news is that only one in twenty thousand eggs carries the salmonella bacterium. And both the FDA and the egg industry have taken steps to make eggs as safe as possible. For example, some brands are pasteurized in their shells to kill salmonella bacteria. (The carton will indicate if the eggs have been pasteurized.) Nonetheless, avoid eating uncooked eggs. Instead of letting your kids lick the bowl—which was always my favorite part of baking—promise them a cookie as soon as the batch comes out of the oven. One more point: A fingerful of cookie dough can contain anywhere from 50 to 110 calories.

HAVE YOUR JUNK FOOD AND EAT IT, TOO

If you're longing for some of these so-called bad carbs but don't want the pounds they might pile on, start thinking and eating creatively. Ask yourself how you can

113

get as much taste with less fat, sugar, and calories. At the same time, if you're not sure about a particular carb indulgence, ask yourself whether it's so good that it's worth wearing! Here are some substitutions to consider.

- **If you crave potato chips, corn chips, or any snack chip, try popcorn instead.** Two ounces of potato chips have 304 calories, 20 grams of fat, 2 grams of fiber, and 365 milligrams of sodium. Three cups of popcorn (unsalted and unbuttered) have 93 calories, 1 gram of fat, 3.5 grams of fiber, and 1 milligram of sodium.
- **If you love pizza as I do, choose a slice with extra veggies instead of high-fat meat toppings.** Two slices of meat pizza contain 600 calories, 24 grams of fat, 3 grams of fiber, and 1,365 milligrams of sodium. Two slices of vegetable pizza contain 360 calories, 12 grams of fat, 3 grams of fiber, and 1,060 milligrams of sodium.

TRUTH

Vegetarians can be fat, too.

To assume that all vegetarians have their weight under control is as absurd as assuming all religious people are virtuous. While it's true that vegetarian diets with a low-fat content and high-fiber foods can be helpful for weight loss, vegetarians—like nonvegetarians—can also make poor food choices, like eating high-fat foods such as whole milk or full-fat cheeses, as well as large amounts of junk (nutritionally empty) foods.

TRUTH

Hunger pangs might simply mean you need water, not food.

Your body often confuses sensations of thirst with hunger. If you've eaten within the last two hours but still feel hungry, try a glass of water rather than a snack. It just might tame your hunger.

- **Should cravings for sugar and fat set in, it may be because your blood sugar and energy are low.** Rather than having a snack cake, choose something with carbs and protein, like peanut butter on apple slices. This choice will stabilize your blood sugar quickly and keep you

TRUTH

Carbs can "comfort" you.

Many people reach for carbs when they are feeling stressed or depressed, leading to weight gain. This isn't surprising, since eating carbohydrates raises levels of serotonin, a mood-elevating chemical in the brain. For good weight control, it's important to know your "comfort carbs," those "trigger" foods that make you lose control (such as pizza, ice cream, or candy bars, for many people). Keep tempting carbs out of sight to manage them sensibly. Or save your comfort-carb foods for a weekly treat. If you give up all your favorite foods, then they'll become forbidden foods and you'll probably end up bingeing on them. Instead of denying yourself, head for the middle of the road.

satisfied longer. The fat in peanut butter is monounsaturated, which is a healthier choice than the processed oils in sugary snack cakes.

- **Enjoy carb-rich foods like doughnuts, most muffins, or croissants as a weekly treat rather than an everyday indulgence.** The rest of the time, choose natural carbs like fruit. Allowing yourself a "treat" food or meal once each week often makes it easier to stick to a healthy diet.

- **When you feel really hungry, reach for "wet" carbs.** Wet carbs, like fruit, veggies, oatmeal, yams, or brown rice, are filled with fiber and moisture and have a "bulk effect" that help curb appetite.

TRUTH

Grapefruit juice doesn't mix with medicines.

As I sit at my desk, I am sipping a little grapefruit juice. Why? I love the taste, and it packs a lot of nutrients. But it could spell trouble for me if I were on certain medications. Unlike other juices, grapefruit inhibits one of the enzyme systems in the intestines; as a result, medicines can become more concentrated. For example, people taking cisapride (for gastric reflux), carbamazepine (for epilepsy and trigeminal neuralgia), or cyclosporine (for rheumatoid arthritis and psoriasis) need to be especially aware of the risk. But because all kinds of prescriptions may be affected— including those for high blood pressure, cholesterol, and angina—the alert is for everyone. Remember to ask your doctor or pharmacist about possible interactions with any medications you're taking.

Hard as it may be to accept, the best diet axiom when it comes to carbs or food in general is "everything in moderation." The trouble with moderation is, to put it mildly, moderation seems dull. But in this era of fanatical diets, moderation ought to be viewed as a beautiful thing, and one of the greatest indulgences.

EXTRA, EXTRA

Lose weight on the cereal diet!

Remember how much Jerry Seinfeld loved cereal on his popular sitcom? Hmmm, he was pretty fit. Maybe he was onto something.

Well, it turns out that eating two cereal meals a day is a great way to lose weight, according to a study of more than one hundred overweight men and women at Purdue University in West Lafayette, Indiana. People who ate one serving of a low-sugar cereal with 2/3 cup skim milk and fruit for breakfast and again either at lunch or dinner for two weeks lost significantly more weight than people who had not.

Of course, there was nothing magical about cereal for fat burning. The secret: Each cereal meal contained about 400 calories, which is less than what most people normally eat at mealtime. In fact, the cereal eaters ate about 500 fewer calories a day than they normally would, resulting in about a pound-a-week weight loss.

There's even more positive news to the cereal-diet story. Cereal may help you shed pounds if you're a late-night eater. Wayne State University scientists in Detroit found that overweight people who ate a bowl of cold cereal with low-fat milk ninety minutes after their evening meal consumed significantly fewer calories during a four-week study than those who did not eat cereal. The reason: The cereal helped eliminate night snacking, a common activity that can really rack up the pounds.

All moderation really means is that you try not to treat yourself poorly, but instead treat yourself well. And you don't deprive yourself of little treats every now and then. You don't need to skip dessert every single day. As long as you don't have a problem such as eating a whole bag of cookies, and you know when to push your "stop button," you may enjoy a few every now and then. Moderation means enjoying some indulgences while knowing there should be limits. So enjoy some carbs. They won't kill you—or your waistline.

Myth #6

Diet Drugs Are a Magic Bullet

In the 1970s, over-the-counter (OTC) diet pills were a rite of passage, and our culture revered the "one pill makes you small" message. OTC diet pills worked for me when I tried them during my chubby days in college. I took them when I got up and before meals. Downing a diet pill instead of a plate of salad sounded to me like an easy way to lose weight.

The pills did curb my appetite and made my body and mind go a little further, faster. I lost weight, but they made my heart skip fast and gave me a dry mouth. Many times I had terrible insomnia. I hated the way I felt. I was miserable, so I quit taking the pills and fought my weight in other ways. Because I hadn't really changed my lifestyle, the pounds crept right back on.

I'm glad I stopped, because the pills weren't safe. It was later discovered that those pills contained a dangerous appetite suppressant called phenylpropanolamine (PPA). PPA can elevate blood pressure and cause hemorrhagic (brain-bleeding) strokes in otherwise healthy, younger people. PPA was yanked off the market in 2000. OTC drug makers immediately changed the ingredients for their drugs, and these products have gone through many such reformulations since. As of today, the newest versions contain caffeine, chromium, ginseng, or other natural ingredients that promise a quick weight-loss fix.

Frankly, I don't know many women and men who haven't tried some pill or another to lose weight. We want desperately to be thinner or more fit. We want to control our eating. We want off the diet roller coaster where we gain 20 pounds, heap on the self-abuse, go on a diet, lose 20 pounds, gain it all back plus another 10. If only there were a magic pill for losing weight, stepping on the bathroom scale would no longer be so depressing. Our January resolution to shed a few pounds would be easier to keep. And the brilliant scientists who developed this magic pill would be richer than God. Scores of diet pills

TRUTH

Fat cells don't go away.

You and I are born with a certain number of fat cells, which generally stays constant. When you gain weight, your body doesn't make more fat cells; your existing fat cells get larger, to as much as six times their minimum size. By contrast, losing weight causes fat cells to shrink and become less metabolically active, but their number goes down only slowly, if at all.

have come and gone, raking in billions of dollars for pharmaceutical companies. Unfortunately, we are no closer to having that magic pill than we were 30 years ago.

ANATOMY OF A MYTH

Weight-loss schemes have a rather raucous history, ranging from wiring jaws shut to the insertion of polyurethane balloons in stomachs to promote fullness, but all have had their shortcomings and failures. The most popular idea is a magic pill that will change brain chemistry, perk up metabolism, and let us part with our pounds quickly.

For a while amphetamine, a drug known on the street as speed, seemed to be that magic pill, until doctors began warning of its severe side effects, which included increased blood pressure and heart rate, a dependency on the drug, and bouts of depression when the pill was withdrawn. Amphetamines are no longer prescribed for weight loss.

Then came fen-phen. The combination of two drugs, phentermine and fenfluramine, seemed to be the answer to many dieters' prayers. Fen-phen and Redux, its close cousin, acted on brain chemistry to control appetite. Dieters clamored for the drugs. Weight-loss clinics sprang up everywhere. Doctors wrote millions of prescriptions a month—many for people who were not overweight and didn't need them. Dieters who wanted to drop only 5 pounds became fans.

But the whole industry collapsed as reports of life-threatening side effects began to filter out. The lungs of some fen-phen patients were destroyed by a fatal disease called primary pulmonary hypertension. Others developed heart valve disease. One hundred sixty people died, and Redux and one of the fen-phen drugs, fenfluramine, were withdrawn from the market. Class-action suits followed, and after billions in payouts, drug makers suffered huge financial losses.

Developing a safe, effective diet pill remains the Holy Grail in obesity treatment. For now, however, no such drug exists. Nonetheless, there are a couple of approved drugs that, under a doctor's guidance, can help you, particularly if you have obesity-related conditions that could be life threatening and you are willing to change your lifestyle.

TRUTH
A little extra protein can help you stay on your diet.

That fish, chicken, steak, or yogurt you enjoy is a natural, bona fide appetite suppressant, one that's safe and works effectively. The truth is, protein adds satiety—the nice feeling of being satisfied after a meal. Satiety may actually reduce your desire to overeat at the next meal. And boosting protein may have other benefits. There is fairly good data that if you eat 25 to 30 percent of your calories from lean protein, it can help you retain lean tissue as you lose weight.

You needn't worry that protein has a downside, either. People think that a high-protein diet is bad for the kidneys. But there's no support for that if you have normal kidney function. I'm certainly not advocating a high-protein diet at the expense of other nutrients, just pointing out that some protein on your plate can be a great weight-control tool.

THE LATEST CROP OF DIET DRUGS

If you have not responded well to a diet and exercise program, your doctor's next line of defense may involve drug therapy to help get your weight under control. As of now, the only two drugs officially approved for use to treat weight loss are the appetite suppressant sibutramine (Meridia) and the "fat blocker" orlistat (Xenical), along with its over-the-counter version, Alli.

They can give you a modest weight loss of about 5 to 20 pounds, usually within the first six months of use. (An amount, by the way, that following a healthy exercise and diet plan could provide without negative side effects.) But none will automatically shrink you back into your college jeans or your wedding tux. These diet drugs work **only** if you also adopt healthier habits, and that still means facing up to the fact that exercise and healthy food must become a part of your life. Let's look briefly at these options and how they work.

Meridia (Sibutramine)

The Skinny: Meridia was approved for use in the United States in 1997 as one of the latest in a new generation of appetite suppressants. It works by increasing the level of serotonin—the chemical in the brain that triggers the pleasure center—and, to a lesser extent, a brain chemical called norepinephrine that is linked to changes in mood. Meridia controls your appetite so that you're less likely to paw around for McDonald's two-for-one coupons in your glove compartment. And the drug does this quite well. According to research: If you follow a reduced-calorie diet while taking this drug, you can typically lose 5 to 8 percent of your weight over six months, on average. That is compared with 1 to 4 percent of weight in dieters following only a diet and taking a placebo (look-alike) pill. If you knock off pounds during the first six months, keep using Meridia and you're likely to keep them off, according to studies, many of them conducted by drug makers. This research hints that Meridia may be a good tool for keeping weight off.

Downside: Meridia can raise blood pressure, increasing the risk of heart attack or stroke. It should not be taken by people with liver or kidney problems. Anyone who takes Meridia should treat it with respect and not as a wonder drug or miracle cure.

Should You Take It? Clearly, Meridia isn't a drug that just anyone can take. It's indicated only if you've been diagnosed as obese (a body mass index [BMI] over 30) or overweight (a BMI over 27), with other risk factors such as diabetes or high cholesterol. By promoting weight loss, Meridia indirectly helps regulate blood sugar and helps keep cholesterol in check. If you're considered overweight, your doctor may prescribe it for you, especially if you have cholesterol and blood sugar problems. You shouldn't take Meridia if you have uncontrolled high blood pressure, heart disease, congestive heart failure, or heart rhythm disturbances or if you are taking other drugs such as antidepressants that increase serotonin levels.

Xenical (Orlistat)

The Skinny: The particular excitement involving Xenical, approved in 1999, hinges on the drug's ability to disable pancreatic enzymes that help the intestines absorb the fat in foods. About 30 percent of the fat in your diet (and the calories in that fat) passes through your digestive tract without being digested or absorbed.

In clinical trials, people taking Xenical lost 9 percent of their body weight in one year, on average, compared with 5.8 percent among those who took a placebo. The drug has also been found to improve blood sugar, cholesterol, and blood sugar control—so it may help prevent heart disease and diabetes if you're at risk.

Taking Xenical may also help you maintain your weight loss. That's no small feat, either, when you consider how tough it is to keep pounds off. Case in point: In long-term studies, people on Xenical regained about 35 percent of their weight during their second year on the medication, while those taking a placebo regained a lot more—about 62 percent.

Downside: As a way to get thin, Xenical has some drawbacks. Fat that isn't absorbed has to go somewhere, and Xenical takers find out in a hurry just where. The oily fat that is not absorbed in your gut can slide right out of you. (Doctors advise keeping an extra pair of pants handy in the event of calamitously embarrassing accidents.) Among the drug's other less elegant side effects are gas with discharge, urgency to have a bowel movement, and fatty or oily stools.

Moreover, about 20 percent of those who take Xenical absorb not only less fat but also fewer nutrients—particularly vitamins D and E and beta-carotene, which is why your doctor will advise you to take a multivitamin daily, at bedtime. To minimize the risk of side effects, it is best to follow a low-fat diet (less than 20 percent or lower of your total daily calories come from fat).

You'll be advised to take Xenical with your three main meals because the drug has to be in your digestive tract when the meals are consumed. It doesn't do much good against between-meal snacks, which are what make many people fat in the first place. And the drug won't work against bad carbs.

Should You Take It? Xenical may be an option for you if you have a BMI of 30 or greater or have a BMI of 27 or greater and have other risk factors, such as high blood pressure, high cholesterol, heart disease, or diabetes. But you should not take it if you just need to drop a few pounds or suffer from disorders of intestinal absorption, inflammatory bowel disease, or blockage of bile flow. The drug can aggravate these conditions.

Alli (Over-the-Counter Orlistat)

The Skinny: I reported on Alli when it became available at drugstores in 2007, no prescription required. With the prescription version (Xenical), up to 30 percent of fat from food is blocked; with the lower-dose OTC formulation, 25 percent of fat is blocked. Alli contains 60 milligrams of orlistat per capsule, taken three times daily with meals; Xenical is prescribed at 120 milligrams three times daily with meals. The amount of fat calories blocked will depend on how much fat you eat, but most patients block 100 to 200 calories per day.

So, how does that play out in pounds? Subjects who took Alli for six months lost 50 percent more weight— say, 15 pounds versus 10—than those who only dieted. If you decide to take Alli alone, without undertaking a weight-loss program, you're going to be disappointed. The drug doesn't work unless you follow a healthy, low-fat diet and do some regular exercise. A starter pack of Alli includes a month's supply of pills, dietary guidelines, a calorie and fat counter, and a food journal.

Downside: If you like your steak, bacon, butter, and other high-fat fare, you're going to have problems with this drug. Eating more than 30 percent of your calories, or roughly 15 grams of fat per meal, can trigger loose, oily stools, since the excess fat that is blocked from absorption is quickly excreted.

Should You Take It? Alli is intended for people who have a BMI of 27 or higher. Some doctors feel that Alli and Xenical are useful for people who eat out often and don't have much control over the amount of fat they are served. However, if you want to lose 5 pounds to fit into your bikini, I suggest that you don't take this drug. Normal-weight people who take Alli place themselves at an unnecessary risk of suffering side effects such as loss of bowel control and vitamin loss. So for the casual dieter, go back to the basics, push yourself away from the table, exercise, and change your lifestyle.

FREE LUNCH? UP-AND-COMING WEIGHT-LOSS DRUGS

Eyeing a potential gold mine in the global obesity epidemic, pharmaceutical companies and universities have launched a massive drive to develop new and better diet pills. And I suspect over the next few years, we'll have ripples of more and more diet drugs hitting the market. After all, the American public is overweight. More than two-thirds of us are obese, and we want something to fix it. Here's a look at the next wave of diet drugs that may soon hit the market, as well as some off-label drugs used to treat obesity.

Rimonabant

Available in Europe since mid-2006 as Acomplia, rimonabant is currently under review by the FDA for prescription use here under the name Zimulti. It has been dubbed the ultimate diet pill and blockbuster drug by the press and medical community. Rimonabant works by blocking endocannabinoid receptors—present in the brain, where they affect cravings, and in fat cells, where they play a role in metabolism. These are the same receptors that bring on the "munchies" in marijuana smokers. Besides helping to control appetite, rimonabant plays a role in the breakdown of glucose and fat, which may explain why people taking the drug see improvement in a range of risk factors for heart disease and diabetes, namely their blood glucose and cholesterol readings, which can't be explained by weight loss alone. Diabetics who took rimonabant for six months lost two and a half times more weight (15 pounds versus 6 pounds) than those taking a placebo, according to a study sponsored by Sanofi Aventis, the drug's manufacturer. As for side effects, people who took rimonabant were slightly more likely to suffer anxiety and depression. Clinically obese people with low levels of high-density lipoproteins ("good" cholesterol) and high levels of triglycerides, who have no history of anxiety or depression, are the best candidates for this drug.

Lorcaserin

Currently in clinical trials, this drug works by activating a serotonin receptor in the brain that helps regulate appetite and metabolism. Early tests demonstrated that lorcaserin produced significant and progressive weight loss over a twelve-week period and was generally well tolerated at all doses. The drug, which hasn't shown safety issues so far, has been under intense scrutiny by analysts who are concerned about its marketing viability, since lorcaserin is said to work similarly to now discontinued fen-phen, which caused heart problems. However, Arena Pharmaceuticals, the company that makes the drug, says lorcaserin is much more selective in the receptors it affects. In clinical trials, the drug had no apparent effects on heart valves or pulmonary artery pressure.

TRUTH

A glass of water before meals helps weight loss.

This is one of my favorite appetite-taming tactics; it gives my stomach a full feeling, so I eat less. Try a clear, brothy soup before a meal, too. It helps outsmart cravings and can tame an out-of-control appetite.

Off-Label Weight-Loss Drugs

Many doctors believe it is sometimes appropriate to prescribe drugs for indications that have not been approved by the FDA—a practice known as off-label use. Off-label use is legal and, with important qualifications, generally embraced by physicians and other health-care providers, health-care institutions, insurers, pharmaceutical companies, and even the FDA. Before prescribing a drug for a use not on the approved label, doctors must be very well informed about the drug, its side effects, and the condition of their patients. Off-label use is not to be undertaken lightly or casually but with wisdom, firm scientific rationale, and sound medical evidence.

So, in our unending quest for a miracle diet pill, Americans are being prescribed an array of prescription drugs approved by the FDA to treat a variety of illnesses. In most cases, the weight-loss side effect of these drugs was a serendipitous finding. People were prescribed the drug for an underlying medical problem, and weight loss was an observed side effect. But none of them has been approved as a diet drug.

The list includes drugs meant to treat attention-deficit hyperactivity disorder (Adderall), depression (Wellbutrin), epilepsy (Topamax and Zonegran), diabetes (Glucophage and Byetta), sleep disorders (Provigil), smoking (Zyban), and even opiate overdoses (Narcan). Often these drugs are used alone, but sometimes they're taken in combination with each other or with popular weight-loss medications.

While there is no hard data on the trend, doctors and patients say it has been increasing for years and that the drugs are being used by Americans, especially women, of all shapes and sizes. Here is where you have to be really careful. Asking your doctor to prescribe an off-label drug for weight loss is medical bungee jumping—and can be risky. I'll use the drug Adderall as an example. Adderall, a stimulant originally marketed as a diet drug in the 1970s under a different name, is now a widely used prescription drug for the treatment of attention-deficit hyperactivity disorder (ADHD). Introduced in 1996 as a treatment for ADHD, Adderall stimulates neurotransmitters in the brain that are believed to improve a person's ability to focus on a given task. One of its major side effects is weight loss, and according to media reports, Adderall is said to be the weight-loss agent of choice for everyone from soccer moms to Hollywood starlets, many of whom take it without a prescription.

Because the drug is an amphetamine, it acts like speed when taken by people who are able to concentrate just fine on their own. The problem with taking a drug like this for a secondary use is that it has side effects that can go far beyond potential weight loss, even when taken as instructed: psychotic episodes, depression, and even serious heart problems. It shouldn't be used casually or frivolously.

It's worth saying again: Weight is best managed by eating a sensible, moderate diet and getting plenty of exercise.

If you're thinking of taking any type of weight-loss drug, discuss your choices and the attendant risk factors with your doctor and decide what course of treatment—including diet and exercise—seems advisable in your situation. You want a program that will help you keep your weight off and not be just a quick fix. Given these drugs' relatively modest effects, the secret of losing weight still lies in what goes into your mouth.

TRUTH

Hormone replacement therapy doesn't prevent weight gain.

If you're a woman going through menopause, you may find it difficult to drop the 5 pounds that was so easy to lose in the past. And watching your calories may not produce the same fast results that you have come to expect. Most, but not all, women gain weight after menopause. Menopause is the process by which estrogen levels decrease as the body undergoes adaptive hormonal changes that will signify the end of fertility. So it would stand to reason that hormone replacement therapy would prevent weight gain, right? Wrong. Hormone therapy seems to have little impact on weight gain. In most studies, women who take estrogen gain the same 4 to 5 pounds as those who avoid postmenopausal replacement.

WHAT ABOUT WEIGHT-LOSS SURGERY?

If even medication fails to work, another resource is bariatric surgery, or weight-loss surgery. It is flourishing. Some 205,000 obesity patients had bariatric surgery in the United States in 2007, when the latest figures were published.

Bariatric surgery is not something you should—no pun intended—take lightly. It is a big endeavor and intended for morbidly obese patients with life-threatening complications from obesity, such as heart disease, high blood pressure, diabetes, and liver problems. Any kind of surgery is stressful—physically, emotionally, and mentally. The more you know about the surgery, the better the chances you will feel at least some sense of control as you proceed with and recover from it. There are two main types of bariatric surgery: gastric bypass surgery and banding surgery. Both procedures alter the gastrointestinal tract to limit the amount of food you can eat.

In gastric bypass (the Roux-en-Y gastric bypass, named for the doctor who invented it), the surgeon creates a small stomach by stapling part of your stomach together. The pouch is about the size of a walnut and limits how much you can eat. Next, a Y-shaped section of the small intestine is attached to the pouch to allow food to bypass the duodenum as well as the first portion of the jejunum. This causes reduced calorie and nutrient absorption.

The surgery has been thrust into the spotlight by celebrity patients, such as the *Today* show's Al Roker, Idol's Randy Jackson, and singer Carnie Wilson. The results can be impressive: Patients typically lose 100 pounds or more the first year when their appetites are almost nonexistent, for reasons doctors can't quite explain. Hypertension and troubles related to joints improve dramatically, and 85 percent of people who have diabetes before surgery see blood sugar levels return to normal.

This operation can also be performed by using a laparoscope—a small, tubular instrument with a camera attached—through short incisions in the abdomen (laparoscopic gastric bypass). The tiny camera on the tip of the scope allows the surgeon to see inside your abdomen.

Compared with the traditional gastric bypass, the laparoscopic technique usually shortens your hospital stay and leads to a quicker recovery. Fewer wound-related problems occur. Not everyone is a candidate for laparoscopic gastric bypass, however. Talk to your surgeon about whether this approach is right for you.

In banding surgery, a band (think thick rubber band) is used to section off a small portion of your stomach to form a small pouch about the size of a golf ball. This restricts the amount of food your stomach can hold, causing you to feel full. Banding surgery is usually reversible. Candidates for both surgeries must be at least 100 pounds overweight with a BMI of more than 40.

I think weight-loss surgery should only be a consideration for people whose obesity puts their lives at risk from hypertension, diabetes, and cardiac problems—and this may include some teenagers who are so obese that they're developing these chronic adult illnesses early. Selected adolescents can benefit from this surgery, but it has to be done at a pediatric center where surgeons tailor surgery to this emerging population group, and don't just treat teens as they would adults. And let me emphasize: Weight-loss surgery is an avenue to be considered only after every attempt has been made to lose weight naturally.

Among the gastric bypass patients I have met is Marietta Sanders, whose experience remains a lesson to anyone considering bariatric surgery. She was thirty-nine years old, single, and had been a real estate broker in San Francisco for many years. Over lunch one day, Marietta told me that she had had a weight problem for as long as she could remember. At 5 feet 4 inches tall and 275 pounds, she was by anyone's definition fat. Marietta—like six million other Americans—fell under the clinical description of morbidly obese, meaning she was more than one hundred pounds overweight.

Like most obese people, Marietta had tried every method of dieting: group diets, liquid diets, herbal diets, fen-phen, and exercise classes. But all her efforts and resolutions failed, and she felt increasingly powerless over the problem. She described how upset it made her feel to be heavy. "As big as we are, we are invisible. People don't look at you, they don't talk to you."

One day, while shopping with her niece, she found that she couldn't walk in the mall without becoming out of breath or feeling pain in her knees. For the first time, she feared for her life—not just the quality of it but the longevity of it.

Marietta was at the end of her rope when she decided to investigate gastric bypass. She read plenty of horror stories: About three persons in a thousand can die from the surgery. Other patients experience serious complications, from bowel obstructions to leaks in their intestines to blood clots. Nonetheless, she decided to take a chance. She headed to a bariatric center in Los Angeles to undergo the surgery. It went well. Over the course of one year, Marietta lost 150 pounds.

Then, as she put it, "I felt invincible. The weight came off so easily I felt I could start eating again to my heart's content." And so she did—whole pizzas, candy bars, cupcakes, chips, cheeseburgers. Of course, this behavior flew in the face of what she was taught during the presurgical education. Even though she experienced the severe nausea and pain that gastric bypass patients get when they overeat or indulge in too many sweets, she kept eating, eating, and eating, no matter how uncomfortable it made her. If she regurgitated the food, that would only make room in her stomach for more food. By not changing her eating habits, Marietta saw her weight balloon back to 275 pounds, with interest. It wasn't that the surgery had failed but that Marietta had failed the surgery.

Marietta is among the 30 percent of patients—the published data conflict on the exact percentage—who regain weight after having a gastric bypass operation. Therein lies the lesson: If you're considering weight-loss surgery, you must be willing to make major changes in your eating habits and lifestyle, postsurgery. Bariatric surgery is not a cure for overeating. Nor is it cosmetic surgery; it's done for health reasons and can be lifesaving—but you still have to change how you eat and how you take care of your body. Without that, you may end up like Marietta.

Anyone considering this surgery should seek an experienced bariatric surgeon rather than someone who does an occasional weight-loss surgery. Just as important, it needs to be performed at centers where there is a comprehensive approach involving surgeons, internists, psychologists, exercise physiologists, and dietitians who can help you forge a lifestyle that supports ongoing weight control.

EXTRA, EXTRA

Eating two eggs for breakfast as part of a reduced-calorie diet can help you lose weight.

Eggs frequently make headlines. Now it turns out they are a great diet food. Eating two eggs for breakfast can help overweight adults lose more weight and feel more energetic than those who eat a bagel containing an equal number of calories, a study reported in the *International Journal of Obesity* shows.

The researchers also found that cholesterol levels were not adversely impacted during the two-month study of 152 overweight individuals. These findings add to more than thirty years of research that conclude healthy adults can enjoy eggs without significantly increasing cholesterol or impacting their risk for heart disease. (Eating eggs isn't really how we get high cholesterol. There are a lot of other culprits in our food supply besides eggs that get turned into cholesterol, namely, fatty meats and dairy.) So you can enjoy an egg several times a week, if you limit cholesterol from other sources—and skip the frying.

As doctors, we truly want effective ways to treat obesity successfully. But I worry that sometimes we look to pills or surgery to fix a problem instead of preventing it from developing. Let's teach our children and teenagers now that these problems can be avoided. The only magic bullet out there: a daily routine that makes exercise and a healthy diet a lifelong habit.

Myth #7

Dieting Is All You Need to Lose Weight

In 2007 I reported on a remarkable experiment conducted in a small town—a battle plan for cities across the United States to fight obesity. The town of note is Somerville, Massachusetts, just two miles north of Boston. Occupying slightly over 4 square miles, Somerville, with its population of eighty thousand, is the most densely populated community in New England.

With its colorful clapboard homes, brick sidewalks, and idyllic street names, Somerville is an eclectic mix of blue-collar families, young professionals, college students, and recent immigrants from countries as diverse as El Salvador, Haiti, and Brazil. Somerville is known for its large number of town squares, which help mark neighborhood boundaries while also featuring bustling businesses and entertainment centers.

There is no lack of history in this New England town.

Note, for example, that Paul Revere galloped through Somerville on the night of April 18, 1775, arousing the farmers to oppose the British on their way to Concord.

Somerville is also the birthplace of Marshmallow Fluff, a smooth, delectable marshmallow crème. Before World War I, a Somerville man named Archibald Query had been making it in his kitchen and selling it door-to-door, but wartime shortages had forced him to close down. By the time the war was over, Mr. Query had other work and was uninterested in restarting his business, but he was willing to sell the formula. Two candy makers and veterans of the U.S. Infantry, H. Allen Durkee and Fred L. Mower, pooled their savings and bought it for $500. They turned the product into the international sensation that it is today.

As in many other cities across America, kids in Somerville are now overweight. But change is under way. More than five years ago, Tufts University researchers Chris Economos and Miriam Nelson enlisted the entire city to attack childhood obesity, not just in schools but in every part of the village. More fruits and vegetables were added to school lunches. Crosswalks even got a fresh coat of paint to encourage walking and biking. The goal of the researchers' plan was to have Somerville children burn more calories through exercise and take in fewer with a healthier diet, for a total deficit of 125 calories a day. The innovative program marked an unusually aggressive response to the growing problem of childhood obesity, which has nearly tripled among U.S. teens during the past two decades.

I was intrigued by the results. After eight months,

students in the first through third grades gained one pound less than students in similar communities. While it may not sound like a lot, this shift in weight gain over time will move many children out of the overweight category.

No part of Somerville daily life was too big or too small to be included. Parents were given homework, newsletters, a monthly column in the local paper—even coupons for healthier food. In school, they implemented huge changes—more whole grains, fruits, and vegetables, taste tests to introduce new foods, nutrition training for teachers and food servers, and ice cream only once a week. After school, students were offered cooking lessons to make healthy snacks.

Even restaurants were involved, making small menu changes such as using low-fat substitutes and offering smaller portions. It didn't hurt that the town's mayor was a health nut and head cheerleader of the experiment. "There was a mind-set that changed toward active living, eating smart, playing hard," the mayor told me.

It wasn't just Somerville's kids who were affected. Parents started exercise and diet programs for themselves, showing that when an entire community comes together, it can be the key to conquering obesity, which is fast overtaking smoking as the country's leading preventable cause of death.

If the town of Somerville could do just two things— get more active and eat more nutritiously—just think what a whole country could do.

ANATOMY OF A MYTH

It is a myth that we can diet our way to slimness, without ever lifting a finger or leg or even a dumbbell—a myth on a par with "lose weight while you sleep," "all-natural fat magnet zaps fat," and other claims that are about as credible as a note from the tooth fairy. These myths have their genesis in quick-fix promises and other diet scams.

As the kids and adults in Somerville learned, you have two major weapons in the battle of the bulge: diet and exercise. They work together to take weight off, and keep it off. Dieting alone might take off weight initially, but you'll gain it back if you're not active. In the same vein, you can work out for hours, but if you live on pizza and ice cream, you may never see those numbers on the scale go down.

There's ample evidence to support this, but one study in particular caught my eye. It analyzed forty-three clinical trials that lasted at least three months and included 3,476 overweight or obese adults who were prescribed a variety of exercises. Researchers found that exercise alone resulted in modest weight loss, compared with no treatment, but people who combined exercise with a low-fat or low-calorie diet lost substantial weight.

Exercise makes some amazing contributions to weight control. One has to do with yo-yo dieting. Let's be honest: Most of us who diet to lose weight have done so more than once. This repeated loss and regain of weight is known as weight cycling, or yo-yo dieting. A typical weight cycle can range from small (i.e., 5 to 10 pounds) to large (i.e., 50 pounds or more) weight losses and gains. If you diet without exercising, your weight will go up and down like a roller coaster.

Your goal with dieting is to jettison extra fat, right? Unfortunately, when you diet without exercise, you will likely lose both fat and muscle. Losing fat is fine, but losing muscle is not, because it slows your metabolism, the chemical process by which our body breaks down food to produce energy. Exercise, particularly strength training, helps preserve muscle that might be otherwise lost when you diet. The more muscle you add to your body through exercise, the higher your metabolic rate will be. By turning your metabolism up a notch, you'll burn more calories even when you're sitting still. And, after vigorous exercise, your caloric expenditure can increase for up to forty-eight hours.

Exercise combined with diet is necessary to make your body selectively lose fat while maintaining (or even increasing) your muscle mass. Muscle makes your body firm, plus endows it with shape. If you're left with some loose skin after dieting, exercising develops muscle that will fill in the slack. You'll begin to see curves where you hadn't before.

There's more: The better-conditioned you are through exercise, the more fat you burn for energy, because your muscles adapt to using an enzyme that oxidizes fat. People who are less trained burn more carbohydrate instead. And exercise can help you with the toughest problem of all: keeping your weight off.

The practical advice here is that you can't rely on exercise alone or diet alone to get trim and fit. The most

TRUTH

It's never too late to start exercising.

Lots of people think they're too old to start an exercise program. They think it's unsafe because they have heart disease, diabetes, or arthritis or because they're too out of shape to start. In one Tufts study, the participants were frail nursing-home residents whose ages ranged from seventy-two to ninety-eight. After just ten weeks, strength-training improved their muscle strength, ability to climb stairs, and walking speed.

The same goes for people with chronic diseases. Exercise can and should be part of the treatment for many diseases. Of course, this doesn't mean that you can plunge into a bout of vigorous exercise, regardless of your health history. You must check with a physician and start at the pace he or she recommends.

effective strategy is to do both—cut calories and increase the amount and intensity of your exercise. If you're overweight and trying to lose weight, exercise is a better ally than any fad diet you may be looking to for help; it should be part of your new lifestyle regimen.

TO YOUR HEALTH .

I must add here that beyond weight control, exercise lowers your risk for many diseases. There is, essentially, no more important activity for the body. Moderate exercise increases the heart's ability to pump blood. Exercise will also decrease the rate at which your heart beats at rest and during moderate exertion.

These two benefits of exercise are absolute. Other benefits include increasing high-density lipoproteins

TRUTH

Men who work out regularly are less likely to have problems with impotence.

Do you want your husband or boyfriend to exercise? Then enlighten him on this truth. It makes sense: Erections depend on blood flow to the penis, so anything that affects the cardiovascular system can wreak havoc on a man's sex life as he ages. How much exercise is enough to make a difference? Enough to burn 200 calories per day, according to a study conducted by the New England Research Institutes.

("good" cholesterol) and decreasing low-density lipoproteins ("bad" cholesterol) and triglyceride levels. Exercise improves the ability of insulin to enter cells, so it lowers the risk of type 2 diabetes. Exercise also improves joint function, decreases the risk for osteoporosis by lessening the loss of bone mineral, keeps you regular, and helps maintain a sense of well-being. Who can argue with such a résumé?

Exercise alters not only your risk for disease, but your quality of life. Exercise improves sleep in people with modest sleep dysfunction, that is, people who take a long time to fall asleep or who wake up frequently at night.

The psychological benefits of exercise are frequently overlooked. Exercise has consistently been shown to relieve depression, stress, and anxiety. Personally, going on a hike or taking a long walk gives me a chance to think through problems; it's the best way to purge everyday stresses that sap stamina. Exercise also raises brain chemicals that energize me.

145

Ever since I started exercising regularly, I've felt better and had more energy—and you know what? If I skip exercising for more than a day or two, I miss it. But I do have to plan it. If you had told me I'd miss exercising ten years ago, I'd have said, you're crazy. But now I know better.

I try to hike and walk most weekends with my husband and children. But during the week, I can't always get away from the house. With the kids here, I've had to figure out how to exercise at home. I keep it simple. I have a treadmill and free weights at home. I admit I have a very short attention span—so I usually work out with the television on or while reading a magazine to keep me from getting bored. I find if the machine's right there I avoid making excuses about not having enough time.

When it comes to exercise, I try to give myself an easy way out—out to exercise, that is. When I travel, I always pack gym shoes. Even if I don't go to the hotel gym, I can walk, and over the years I've stuck to my walking regime better than I have to any other out-of-town workout.

If you're feeling overwhelmed by the prospect of adding an exercise program to your already hectic life and if you're feeling defeated by years of inactivity, don't say, "Oh well, I've lost that battle." Start with small steps. Any amount of exercise you can add to your daily routine will help maintain your health.

I was on television with Martina Navratilova recently and reminded her about advice she gave people years ago. After she immigrated to the United States, her weight ballooned. One reason was that she ate a lot of ice cream without burning it off. She was in the dumps and trying to find the source of her unhappiness. Martina made a list for herself: the things she liked about herself in the first column and the things she didn't in the second. Much to her surprise, she put almost all of her qualities in the plus column and only one in the negative column: her weight. So she set about changing it.

A big part of her strategy was to increase her physical activity with things she enjoyed. Martina says, "Find your passion, and whatever it is, do it, whether it's walking or playing softball. Just move your body. You don't have to be an elite athlete to get fit, either." Martina also pointed out that the more fit you become, the more you can walk past the doughnuts and choose fresh fruit instead.

TRUTH

A combination of aerobic exercise and strength training is the best workout for weight loss.

I used to think that the more cardio I did, the more fat I'd lose. Now I know that you need a combination of aerobic exercise and strength training to burn fat and keep it off. Aerobic exercise can help you become more cardio fit and create a deficit of calories faster than resistance training, but strength training helps by maintaining muscle mass. Muscle mass is imperative for a strong metabolism, and for keeping your metabolism fast—and that is key to fat loss. The more lean muscle you have, the more fat you burn, even when you are at rest. That doesn't mean you have to look like a bodybuilder to be an efficient fat-burning machine. But you do have to at least maintain and preferably increase your lean muscle mass. So in a nutshell, a combination of properly monitored aerobic exercise and resistance training enables you to rapidly burn the maximum amount of fat.

Exercise strengthens not only your body but also your resolve to get in better shape and enjoy better health. Martina knew that if she could accomplish so many positive things in her life, she could conquer her weight problem, too. She figured it out; so can you.

So, if you don't yet have a regular exercise program, try to develop one. And as ever, consult your doctor before doing so. If you've had trouble sticking to an exercise program in the past, read on for more motivation.

TAKING ACTION

A lot of people regard exercise as something like climbing Mount Everest—you've got to get there first, you need a lot of equipment, and the goal is almost insurmountable and relentlessly time consuming. Of course, nothing could be further from the truth. No, really. Here's the scoop on some easy ways to get started and stick with it.

Keep It Simple and Enjoyable

Exercise can be as simple and pleasant as a long, brisk walk on the beach or around the block. All you have to do is get out there and walk, and keep a decent pace. Or go to the gym and walk on the treadmill, listening to music. Don't be overwhelmed by all the media hype that might make you think you're not exercising unless you're playing professional basketball. That's not the point. The point is to keep your body moving, to get your heart to an aerobic level of activity at least three times a week for

TRUTH

Exercising with improper form burns fewer calories.

You may not realize it, but you could be subtly sabotaging your workout by exercising with improper form—and burning fewer calories as a result. When exercising on a stair climber or treadmill, keep your back straight and weight centered. Leaning on the handles of cardio equipment puts you at risk of back or knee injury and makes you burn about 25 percent fewer calories than the machine's display says you are.

twenty to thirty minutes, and to make exercise a part of your life. There are lots of choices, too. Find something you enjoy. There is dancing, swimming, biking, hiking, ice skating, playing golf . . . There is no reason to say no. Put your mind in neutral and enjoy yourself.

Sneak Exercise In

Don't underestimate the value of everyday activities like housework and gardening for burning calories. That's how our moms and grandmothers kept fit! Can these "lifestyle activities" really do the same for us? Some very convincing research says yes. One of these studies, conducted by researchers at the Cooper Institute for Aerobics Research, compared the twenty-four-month effects of a lifestyle activity program with traditional structured exercise on improving physical activity, cardiorespiratory fitness, and cardiovascular disease risk factors on 235 sedentary adults (116 men and 119 women). The researchers found that both groups significantly improved their cardiovascular fitness and blood pressure, plus lost body fat.

Putting more action into your day is a simple way to burn more calories. Let's say you vacuum your house three times a week, for an hour each time. You use up to 480 calories a week. That might not seem like much, except in a year you've expended 24,960 calories, or 7 pounds.

Ask yourself: "Do I need a car for this errand or can I walk?" So many ordinary everyday activities count as moderate-intensity exercise: walking instead of driving, cutting the lawn with a push mower, or playing with the children. All of these activities burn calories. See the chart on page 159 for different activities that can help you drop pounds almost automatically.

Another key is to move around more. Squirming in your seat, tapping your toes, and generally changing your posture frequently can account for a significant portion of the calories burned in a day, anywhere from 15 percent in a sedentary person to 50 percent in someone who is very active, scientists at the Mayo Clinic have found. In an eight-week study, sixteen volunteers were fed the equivalent of two large burgers a day on top of their normal food needs, while doing very little exercise.

Their weight gains were measured and the scientists discovered that the people who had fidgeted the most were the ones who had suffered the smallest increase. The scientists found that for every 1,000 extra calories consumed by the volunteers, 39 percent ended up as fat, but up to 33 percent was burned off by NEAT (nonexer-

TRUTH

Pedometers inspire greater calorie burning.

As a medical reporter, I'm on my feet for eight to ten hours during the day. I once wore a pedometer and learned I walked more than 11,000 steps (that's over 5 miles) in one day! This is why I now recommend wearing a pedometer to track your daily steps. (You can find a pedometer for $20 to $60 at gyms and sporting goods stores.) It also helps you make better decisions through the day. You begin to learn that little things do add up.

Ultimately, aim for at least 10,000 steps a day. That's a safe and effective goal for most people, although 12,000 steps a day are better for weight loss. Adding 2,000 steps a day—the equivalent of walking approximately 1 mile—burns about 80 extra calories.

cise activity thermogenesis), or, in layman's terms, fidgeting. So basically, people with the greatest increase in NEAT gained the least fat and those who had the least change in NEAT gained the most fat. NEAT could explain why some people don't gain weight, even when they overeat. The moral of the story: If you want to avoid

TRUTH

Exercising doesn't mean you can eat anything you want.

It's a lot easier to eat calories than burn them. Eat one cheeseburger and you'll cancel out the 350 calories you burned in a forty-five-minute exercise class.

extra body fat, move around like a little kid with ants in his or her pants. Constant fidgeting could be the secret to weight loss.

Find the Time

Like everyone else's, my life is a busy one. With so much to accomplish each day, I deliberately walk first thing in the morning, before most people have left their warm beds. This time of the day works best for me, too, because I've usually run out of steam by the evening.

Look at your own schedule and determine where you can regularly fit in a thirty-minute exercise session. For some people, this may mean getting up a half-hour earlier. For others, lunchtime or after work is most convenient. Your goal is to improve your health and lose pounds by doing thirty minutes or more of an activity that's moderately intense, five days a week. If you don't reach this goal at first, it's good to remember that any increase in physical activity is better than none.

Break It Up

A significant plus for busy people is that activity doesn't have to be done in a single session. You can break up the thirty minutes—for example, by taking a ten-minute walk to the store and later having a twenty-minute bike ride with the kids. There's ample evidence to show that breaking up physical activity into ten-minute spurts throughout the day burns up at least as many calories as exercising in a single block of time. Once you get into

TRUTH

Working out seven days a week can make you less efficient.

Overdoing it can leave you exhausted, strain joints and muscles, and weaken your immunity. Rest is just as important as working out because muscles need time to repair, so schedule some time off from exercising, even if it's just one day. Change things up a bit, too, with "cross-training," or engaging in more than one type of physical activity to avoid the overuse of one set of muscles: weights one day, cardio the next, followed by a day of rest.

the habit of setting aside time on most days, you'll be more open to new kinds of activities—because you'll feel stronger and more capable of exerting yourself. If you've never considered taking up a new sport, you might find yourself wielding tennis racquets, strapping on cross-country skis, or joining a recreational volleyball team. Becoming more active over time helps the effort to keep pounds off.

TRUTH

Muscle does not turn into fat if you stop exercising.

Firm, toned muscles may degenerate into soft, mushy muscles, but they won't turn into fat. Muscle cells and fat cells are two completely different tissues and neither can ever turn into the other.

TRUTH

Spot reduction will not help flatten your stomach.

"Spot reduction" is targeted exercise believed to reduce fat stores in certain "trouble areas" of the body. The theory is that if you exercise a specific area or muscle group, more fat will be burned from that area. As attractive as this sounds, increasing a muscle's activity doesn't burn off fat in that area. Sorry for the bad news, but spot reduction belongs in fairy tales.

You can, however, burn the fat by walking, jogging, running, or other forms of aerobic exercise. Aerobic exercise, as well as strength training, does a good job of triggering the release of belly fat. Combine aerobics with crunches and sit-ups to firm the underlying muscle, and you'll have a great-looking six-pack.

Get a Pet

I'm serious. Walking your dog is exercise. Having a pet lowers stress and is good for your immune system. People who own pets report being happier and it will get you out of the house.

Up the Beat

Focus at first on aerobic activities or exercises that make your heart and lungs work harder. These include walking, jogging, swimming, cycling, dancing, gardening, playing racquetball, and a host of other activities. Then aim for at least thirty minutes of activity in a day. If you can do it all at once, great. But remember, three ten-minute

TRUTH

Huffing and puffing can be a sign you're working out too hard.

How can you tell if you're exercising too hard? What I do is apply the "talk test" to my workouts: If I can't say a sentence or two without completely losing my breath, then I'm exercising too hard and I should decrease my intensity. But if I can carry on a somewhat breathless conversation, then I know I'm at the right intensity.

bursts of activity are fine, too. Don't hesitate to go beyond that thirty-minute target—the longer you are active, the more you benefit.

Get Strong

Toning, stretching, and strength building should be a part of your exercise program as you age, since keeping your joints healthy and staying limber are both important in defending yourself against the wear and tear of aging on the bones, joints, and muscles. I love free weights. Not only do they make the muscles fit, but since they also strengthen bones, posture improves, too. I don't keep my weights in one place, either. They're spread all over the house. When I see them, I pick them up and start pumping.

Women: The weights don't have to be heavy and you don't have to worry about adding bulk to your frame. Plenty of data shows that if you lift weights, no matter

TRUTH

Muscle doesn't weigh more than fat.

A pound of muscle and a pound of fat weigh the same, a pound, just as a pound of feathers and a pound of rocks weigh one pound each. What most people don't realize is that a pound of muscle is denser and takes up less space than a pound of fat. Therefore, having more developed muscle on your frame with less body fat will make you look leaner and more toned. One pound of muscle also burns more calories than 1 pound of fat. Estimates indicate that one pound of muscle burns roughly 50 calories per day, while 1 pound of fat burns approximately 2 calories per day.

what your age, your muscles and bones get stronger. So add some weight lifting or other resistance exercises to your aerobic activities. Choose weights that let you do 12 to 15 repetitions of exercises that work your arm, leg, shoulder, back, and glute muscles.

TRUTH

Exercising to the point of pain can cause injury.

When I feel a little burning in my thighs during an uphill hike, that's a healthy response from my muscles to working hard. Even the muscle soreness I get the next day is okay; it's not a sign that I've injured myself. It's just a sign that I exerted myself. Pain is something else entirely. If what you feel during exercise isn't muscular (there's a sharp pain in your knees or a twinge in your back), stop at once. Exercise should not cause this type of pain. Nor should you try to push through pain when working out.

Limber Up

Exercises such as Pilates, yoga, and gentle stretches are wonderful for your muscles, mind, and overall health. Of course, they can also improve your balance and flexibility. Regular flexibility training helps reduce your risk of injury, improves your mobility, and is a very important part of a healthy, active lifestyle. Balance is absolutely crucial for performing day-to-day activities but diminishes markedly with age—as much as 75 percent from age 25 to age 75—and this increases the risk of falls. People whose balance is poor are often afraid of falling and this interferes with the quality of their lives. Fortunately, balance can be learned and improved through various types of exercises, including yoga and sports.

You know this from learning how to ride a bike or ice skating—examples of challenges to equilibrium that are mastered in exactly the same way a baby learns to sit, crawl, walk, and run. Most people skip flexibility training

TRUTH

Your greatest fitness gains come in the first few weeks of starting an exercise program.

If you're just beginning an exercise program, you should notice changes within the first six weeks. After that, results are cumulative. This means the longer you continue to work out, the more benefits you will see. You'll see even more changes by the third month as long as you keep at it.

because they think it doesn't have a direct impact on their weight. But without proper stretching you could become injured, thus missing many workouts and unable to meet your fitness and weight goals.

The research is clear—nothing improves life and life expectancy more than exercise. So do it. You'll feel better. And don't consider it a choice. Just start slowly and work your way up. Remember, it's not only what you eat, but that you move.

EXTRA, EXTRA

Popping a nonprescription painkiller and lifting weights builds muscle in your quads.

If you're a fit older adult, that is. In a three-month study of people ages 60 to 78, lifting weights regularly and taking daily doses of ibuprofen (like that in Advil) or acetaminophen (like that in Tylenol) led to substantially greater increases over inactive placebo in quadriceps muscle mass and strength. The dosages were identical to those recommended by the manufacturers and were selected to most closely mimic what chronic users of these medicines were likely to be taking.

Resistance training alone (placebo group) increased quadriceps muscle mass and muscle strength. However, the muscles of the ibuprofen and acetaminophen users got 40 to 60 percent bigger than the placebo group's and their muscle strength also went up higher than the placebo group's.

Why did painkillers boost mass and strength? These pills triggered changes within the muscle that enhanced the metabolic response to resistance exercise, allowing the body to add substantially more new protein to muscle.

CALORIES BURNED PER HOUR IN COMMON ACTIVITIES

Aerobic exercise	422
Bicycling	563
Bicycling, stationary	493
Circuit training, gym	563
Cleaning house	246
Dancing	317
Fishing	281
Fixing dinner	176
Gardening	352
Golf, using a cart	246
Jogging	493
Moving furniture	422
Mowing your lawn (not with a riding mower)	387
Playing with your kids, light activity	176
Repairing your car	211
Snorkeling	352
Stair climber–type exercise	422
Sweeping your sidewalk	281
Swimming freestyle	563
Tennis	493
Wallpapering	317
Yoga	281

Adapted from www.nutristrategy.com

EXTRA, EXTRA

Strength training alters bad eating habits.

Want to eat better, automatically? Start pumping iron! A study by Brigham Young University researchers, published in the *Journal of the American Dietetic Association,* found that women who lifted weights three times a week for three months reduced their fat intake to 30 percent of total calories because they became more health conscious as a result of working out.

Myth #8

Supplements Will Make You Thin and Healthy

During my thirty years as a medical reporter, I have interviewed actors, actresses, musicians, teachers, doctors, bankers, professional athletes, Nobel laureates, Somali warlords, movers and shakers, and ordinary people who have done extraordinary things. Add to that list a blue man. And I don't mean a guy who was "depressed," nor do I mean a guy from the popular Blue Man group.

I mean a middle-aged man who is as blue as a Smurf.

Distrustful of doctors, this guy started drinking a dietary supplement called colloidal silver ten years ago after seeing an ad for it in a magazine. Colloidal silver is a suspension of silver in a liquid base. Telling his story on the *Today* show in 2008, he claimed it "cured" several chronic conditions he had, including sinus problems, arthritis, and acid reflux. After he put it on his face to treat a severe case of dermatitis, his skin turned blue—a condition known medically as argyria. With argyria, the silver deposits itself in the skin and other organs and does not go away. Silver is a heavy metal, and it can collect in the organs and cause kidney and liver damage and even brain seizures.

Silver has antibacterial properties, and it has been used to fight infection for thousands of years. But it went out of use when penicillin, which is far more effective, was developed. Nonetheless, it is still sold as a dietary supplement. Marketers claim that colloidal silver benefits the immune system; kills disease-causing agents such as bacteria, viruses, and fungi; offers an alternative to prescription antibiotics; and treats diseases such as cancer, human immunodeficiency virus, acquired immunodeficiency syndrome, tuberculosis, syphilis, scarlet fever, shingles, herpes, and pneumonia. These claims have not been proven.

On air, I urged him to get a medical exam to make sure the silver solution had not damaged his organs. His case of the blues is permanent, by the way. Even if he stopped taking colloidal silver, his skin color would not return to normal. Our blue man came back to the *Today* show after taking my advice and getting a checkup from a cardiologist at St. Luke's–Roosevelt Hospital in New York. The cardiologist reported that he was in good physical condition, but a report was still pending on the silver levels in his organs and whether they would cause long-term damage.

Besides argyria, other side effects of taking colloidal silver include neurologic problems (e.g., seizures), kidney damage, stomach distress, headaches, fatigue, and skin irritation. In addition, colloidal silver may interfere with the body's absorption of prescription medications, including penicillin, quinolones, tetracyclines, and thyroxine.

There is really no reason to take colloidal silver. There's no science behind it, and I worry about its safety. The FDA has taken action against a number of companies for making druglike claims about this type of product.

The issue of nutritional supplementation is difficult to ignore when Americans spend an estimated $22 billion a year on supplements, according to *Nutrition Business Journal.* Such a staggering figure is proof that people believe supplements can replace not only food but also sound medicine. I do not mean to be a killjoy on dietary supplements, but these days, more negative science on them is crossing my desk than ever before.

Case in point: During the first half of 2008, the FDA received 604 "adverse-event" reports—a list that included five deaths—for the use of food supplements. An adverse event can be anything from a concern that a supplement isn't working to a serious illness that follows ingestion of one. An FDA spokesman said that some of these deaths were likely due to underlying medical conditions, exacerbated by taking certain supplements.

The FDA did not identify which supplements were at fault. But they could have been any of the substances defined by the agency as supplements, including vitamins; minerals; herbs or other botanicals; amino acids; and substances such as enzymes, organ tissues, glandulars, and metabolites. Dietary supplements can also be extracts or concentrates and may be found in many forms such as tablets, capsules, softgels, gelcaps, liquids, or powders. They come in other guises, too, such as nutrition bars. Whatever their form, the government places dietary supplements in a special category under the general umbrella of "foods," not drugs, and requires they be labeled as dietary supplements.

TRUTH

We have great science on many dietary supplements.

Numerous studies are published each year in major medical journals that document new findings about whether dietary supplements work and how they might be used to address specific conditions, reduce the risk of diseases, or enhance general nutrition. Such studies can be found in the *Journal of the American Medical Association,* the *New England Journal of Medicine,* the *American Journal of Cardiology,* the *American Journal of Clinical Nutrition,* and the *Journal of the National Cancer Institute.* The information gleaned from these studies has greatly added to our knowledge regarding the effectiveness of commonly used supplements.

Another place to find reliable, unbiased information on supplements is ConsumerLab.com, the website of an independent research organization that tests supplements. There is a yearly subscription to the site, which posts all of the lab's product reports. In some instances, supplements tested by ConsumerLab have been found to contain ingredients not printed on their labels. A recent test of weight-loss supplements, for example, found that some were contaminated with lead. More often, though, the lab discovers what's not in the supplement.

ANATOMY OF A MYTH

In ever-increasing numbers, Americans are embracing self-medication: a do-it-yourself approach to health care that favors home-designed, prevention-oriented supplement regimens. Six out of every ten people in the United States pop nutritional supplements—a trend that dates back to the nineteenth and early twentieth centuries when America was inundated with "patent medicines," that is, suspect remedies that promised to cure seemingly every affliction known to humankind, from indigestion to paralysis to "female troubles." Popular patent medicines, which promised miraculous results, were readily available at general stores and even from seed merchants. Some were also sold by "snake oil salesmen" out of the backs of wagons, with claims of instant cures backed up by convincing testimonials from paid performers.

The contents of these concoctions were jealously guarded secrets and often included hefty concentrations of alcohol. Opium, cocaine, and other addictive substances were not uncommon ingredients. So it's not too surprising that many customers not only experienced relief of their pain and other complaints but also had a strong urge to keep taking the wonder potions. Patent medicines were mostly quackery and provided little lasting benefit. Indeed, with the exception of purgatives like Ex-Lax and Phillips' Milk of Magnesia, few have persisted.

Passage of the Pure Food and Drug Act in 1906 marked the beginning of the end of patent medicines.

Even so, the hucksterism of the industry somehow survives today in the marketing of dubious nutritional therapies that promise, among other modern-day miracles, weight loss, "male enhancement," and almost every other imaginable cure.

Good dietary supplements are exactly what they say—a supplement that "adds to" something. They add to a good diet but can't replace one. Fruit and vegetables contain a spectrum of nutrients, fiber, and phytochemicals that pills can never duplicate. Dietitians believe that vitamins and minerals are vital to good health, but that they work better when eaten whole in foods. Some experts caution that "mega-dosing" on certain vitamins or minerals can displace other nutrients, defeating the original purpose of taking vitamins to improve health.

TRUTH

Energy bars aren't healthier than real food.

Manufactured foods such as energy bars are a good idea at appropriate times and places, and they can be used in a weight-loss program. But don't think of them as "better" than a meal made of whole foods such as fruits, vegetables, and lean proteins. Nutrition bars and other streamlined foods are convenient, but many have a lot of refined sugars and milk fats and contain very little fiber. For your snacks, a better bet is to focus on foods that contain both protein and healthy carbs. Try raisins and nuts or cottage cheese and fruit, either of which can give you protein, iron, and fiber. They also can give you an energy boost for far less money.

Also, many preparations simply don't do what their makers imply. Companies seize on a few shreds of evidence that an herb, nutrient, or whatever will treat or prevent a disease, and then they promote it as a cure-all.

But what takers of many of these supplements aren't seeing is that every few months or so, well-done studies cast doubt on the use of particular supplements. Consider the misfortunes of these remedies in recent years.

Beta-carotene. This substance took a hit several years ago when Finnish smokers, taking it as a supplement in a large trial, seemed to have a higher incidence of cancer than those not taking it. Similar results from the Beta-Carotene and Retinol Efficacy Trial also suggested that this is not a supplement smokers want to ingest. Results from the Physicians' Health Study showed *no* benefits from taking it to healthy people.

Vitamin A. High doses (more than 10,000 international units daily) might cause birth defects, according to Boston University researchers.

Vitamin E. Once thought to be good for the heart, vitamin E taken in amounts of 400 international units or more daily for longer than one year increased the risk of death. Experts now say adults shouldn't take vitamin E preparations in amounts of 400 international units or more, if at all.

TRUTH

Vitamin C does not protect against the common cold.

People still rush for vitamin C at the first sniffle. But does it fight the common cold or even keep germs at bay? Not really, unless you run marathons, are a skier, or are a soldier on a subarctic exercise. For the rest of us, vitamin C can be harmful when taken in large doses over long periods of time. It can produce diarrhea, which can be dangerous in children and elderly people.

Selenium. Until recently, it was thought that the mineral selenium was worth taking as a supplement. Not only is it an antioxidant, meaning that it prevents a rustlike process called oxidation from damaging cells, it also was believed to improve the way the body handles sugar and to possibly prevent some complications of diabetes. But in a large study designed to test whether selenium (200 micrograms daily) could prevent skin cancer, it instead appeared to raise the risk of diabetes. More people who took selenium developed diabetes than those who took a placebo.

Multivitamins. Men who pop too many multivitamins, defined as taking multivitamins more than seven times a week, in the hope of improving their health may in fact be raising their risk of advanced prostate cancer by about 30 percent. This was particularly true in men with a family history of the disease. This was a big study, too: Some 295,344 men were followed over five years to see if there was a link between multivitamin use and prostate cancer. The researchers didn't see any link with an increase of prostate cancer overall; the increased risk from overuse of multivitamins was tied to metastatic prostate cancer or cancer that proved fatal.

Ephedra. This herb was banned in 2004 (after a lengthy court fight) because the weight-loss ingredient increases the risk of heart attack and stroke. The prior year, I remember reading about one of these deaths—the heat-stroke death of twenty-three-year-old Baltimore Orioles pitcher Steve Bechler, which a medical examiner believed was at least partly caused by an ephedra supplement he took.

Other Supplements. In 2004 the Consumers Union, the independent nonprofit publisher of *Consumer Reports,* warned Americans that they should avoid a "dirty dozen" of supplements that may cause cancer, heart problems, kidney or liver damage, even death. On the list were aristolochic acid (snakeroot), comfrey, androstenedione, chaparral, germander, kava, bitter orange (citrus aurantium), over-the-counter organ/glandular extracts (thought to increase the risk of mad cow disease, particularly from brain extracts), lobelia, pennyroyal oil, skullcap, and yohimbe.

I know you read this and think, Darn, why is it all so complicated? But the best response to all the confusion is for us to eat our vitamins and minerals: eat real, healthy food. Eat those brussels sprouts, broccoli, and other good-for-you foods. Our bodies need nutrients for

TRUTH

Antioxidant supplements do not prevent cancer and heart disease.

Before you gulp down handfuls of antioxidant supplements, consider this: They may not be good for you. An analysis of forty-seven studies involving more than 180,000 participants taking beta-carotene, vitamin E, and vitamin A indicated that rather than improving health, popping those pills may increase the risk of death. The report appeared in the *Journal of the American Medical Association* and was compiled by researchers with the Cochrane Collaboration, an international network of experts who conduct systematic reviews of published studies to determine whether current treatments are based on scientific evidence.

Vitamin C and selenium were also included in the analysis and no increased risk of death was found. But people taking vitamin C didn't necessarily live any longer than people who didn't take the vitamin. Although antioxidant supplements are not recommended, antioxidant food sources— especially plant-derived foods such as fruits, vegetables, whole-grain foods, and vegetable oils—are your best bets for good health.

growth, digestion, and other functions. There just isn't any substitute for the nutrients you obtain directly from the food you eat. If you're expecting to make up for a nutrient-poor diet of junk food and black coffee with a handful of supplements, forget it. It doesn't work, and it may make you worse off than the junk would on its own.

THE TEN MOST POPULAR SUPPLEMENTS

SUPPLEMENTS	PRO/CON COMMENTS
1. Multivitamins/minerals	Most people can benefit from taking a multiple daily to fill in any nutritional gaps. These supplements, however, are not meant to "cure" diseases.
2. Sports nutrition powders / formulas	For athletes, these products are helpful in endurance events for quick fueling in a race. Though fairly economical and extremely convenient, sports nutrition products aren't truly necessary for an athlete's regimen. Training effects, such as muscle recovery, can be achieved with real food.
3. Calcium	Supplementing with calcium is recommended, particularly for menopausal women, to protect against osteoporosis. Calcium may also protect against cancer of the colon.
4. B vitamins	Most well-conducted trials of folic acid / vitamin B supplementation have shown that they confer no protection against heart disease, stroke, or cognitive decline.
5. Vitamin C	Supplementing with vitamin C has no effect on longevity of colds, according to recent studies on antioxidants. In doses exceeding the daily recommended dietary allowance, supplemental vitamin C may have a harmful effect on the immune system.
6. Glucosamine/chondroitin	Glucosamine and chondroitin sulfate are natural substances found in healthy joint cartilage. Both are used as alternative treatments to help osteoarthritis. Research is mixed. Both supplements hold promise for moderate to severe knee osteoarthritis; however, a 2008 study published in the *Annals of Internal Medicine* found that taking 1,500 milligrams of glucosamine daily for two years did not help relieve pain, increase daily function, or reduce joint space narrowing in patients with hip osteoarthritis. High dosages (above what is recommended) of glucosamine may cause gastric problems, nausea, diarrhea, indigestion, and heartburn.
7. Homeopathy	Homeopathy is based mostly on the principle that "like cures like" (that which you have is that which I will give you in tiny doses—similar to the principle behind most vaccines).

SUPPLEMENTS	PRO/CON COMMENTS
7. Homeopathy (*continued*)	Supporters say that homeopathy is safe and often helpful, so gold-standard proof is unnecessary; others are not so convinced. Large, systematic studies have failed to show its effectiveness for any condition.
8. Other vitamins	If you've been taking vitamin supplements in hopes of preventing cancer, save your money. The National Institutes of Health found that isolated dosages of synthetic vitamins did nothing to help subjects ward off cancer. While some observational studies have suggested that vitamin takers have lower rates of cardiovascular disease, it isn't clear if this is due to the supplements. For example, supplement users may be taking care of their health in other ways and be less overweight and more physically active.
9. Fish oils	The American Heart Association recommends that patients with documented heart disease take about 1 daily gram of EPA + DHA (eicosapentaenoic acid and docosahexaenoic acid, respectively, types of omega-3 fatty acids), preferably from fish, although EPA + DHA supplements could be considered, but consult with your doctor first.
	For people with high triglycerides (blood fats), 2 to 4 grams of EPA + DHA per day, in the form of capsules and administered under a physician's care, are recommended.
10. Coenzyme Q10	Coenzyme Q10 is a popular antioxidant widely used to treat heart failure, cancer, migraines, and aging. Most investigators conclude that additional research is needed before its use can be recommended medically.

Source: Adapted from Nutrition Business Journal 2007 survey.

HOW TO DEVELOP A RESPONSIBLE SUPPLEMENT STRATEGY

I'm not saying that all supplements are worthless or harmful. They have their place. While a well-balanced and varied diet will take you far, even if you have a stellar diet, it's tough to get optimal amounts of certain nutrients, such as vitamin D. Our food supply isn't what it used to be, and most people don't buy fresh produce from their local farmers anymore. The vegetables you buy at your supermarket might be a week old or more before they reach the store. And, even under the best of circumstances, vitamin and mineral levels in foods are dependent on highly variable growing conditions. Plus, who can honestly say that they eat a perfect diet all the time? For dietary insurance, and to keep things simple, I'm comfortable recommending a daily vitamin / mineral supplement—and eating lots of fresh fruits and vegetables. As for what type of vitamin/mineral to choose, it's a good idea to go with one formulated by a pharmaceutical company to ensure quality. And look for *USP* on the label. This means that the supplement meets the standards of the United States Pharmacopeia (USP). USP is an organization that sets standards for content, quality, purity, and safety. Supplementation isn't an either–or situation; eat the best you can, and take a multiple to fill in possible gaps.

I do have to add that at certain life stages, you may require more of a particular nutrient than your diet can serve, such as folic acid for women of childbearing age, or calcium for pregnant and nursing women. Here is some science-based advice to help you.

Boning Up: Calcium

Calcium's most important function is maintaining bone strength, but it also plays a role in blood clotting and muscle/nerve function. Every cell in your body needs calcium to work properly. Maintaining an adequate calcium intake is an important step toward good bone health throughout life. Luckily, there are many foods that contain calcium. The best sources of calcium include milk, yogurt, and cheese, but you can also get calcium from spinach, soy milk, tofu, almonds, broccoli, oranges, bread, fortified ready-to-eat cereals, fortified fruit juice, and canned salmon with bones.

During the different stages in our lives, our bodies have different needs for calcium. Here is the breakdown of calcium recommendations for different ages for both females and males that you should try to get from food first.

- 1 to 3 years of age: 500 milligrams per day
- 4 to 8 years of age: 800 milligrams per day
- 9 to 18 years of age: 1,300 milligrams per day
- 19 to 50 years of age: 1,000 milligrams per day
- 51 years and older: 1,200 to 1,500 milligrams per day

If you can't meet these recommendations through food, talk to your doctor about supplements. As for the type of calcium supplement to take, calcium carbonate and calcium citrate are the most easily absorbed combinations. Make sure you take calcium in concert with vitamin D, which helps the body better absorb the mineral. Here is a big exception to all this: Men should not take supplemental calcium, since some research suggests excessive calcium may increase the risk for prostate problems. While there is debate regarding how worthwhile supplements may be, there is no debate about the importance of supplemental calcium if you are a woman.

Vitamin B_{12} as You Age

Vitamin B_{12} is needed for nerves and red blood cells, to help develop genetic materials in the cells, and to prevent some forms of anemia. This vitamin is present in almost all animal products. Good sources include flounder, sardines, herring, liver, poultry, eggs, and milk. It needs to be broken down, however, and that process is less efficient as we age. If you're over age fifty, try to get 2.4 micrograms of vitamin B_{12} daily. Most multivitamins provide at least 2.0 micrograms. Also, vegetarians who eat neither eggs nor dairy products might have a tough time consuming enough vitamin B_{12} and may need to supplement.

Iron Rx

Iron is an important mineral during pregnancy for both mother and developing child, which is why iron supplements are often recommended for pregnant women who are deficient in this mineral. If you're a woman of childbearing age who may become pregnant, eat foods high in "heme iron," the easily absorbed animal-source form of the mineral found in lean meats. Whole-grain cereals, beans, and dark leafy vegetables are good iron sources, too, though the iron is not as well absorbed. Eating plant sources of iron in tandem with foods high in vitamin C (such as peppers and citrus fruits) increases iron absorption. Most people do not need to supplement with extra

TRUTH

Spinach is not a great source of iron.

Despite what Popeye led a lot of young people to believe, spinach is not particularly rich in iron. In reality, it has about the same iron content as any other green vegetable. Spinach also contains oxalic acid, which prevents more than 90 percent of the iron from being absorbed by the body. But spinach is a rich source of vitamin A, vitamin E, and several vital antioxidants, with more than a half-day supply of beta-carotene found in just a half cup of the vegetable. (The idea that spinach contains exceptional levels of iron originated in 1870 with scientists whose figures remained unchallenged until 1937, when it was discovered that the content was one-tenth the claim. The oversight resulted from a misplaced decimal point.)

iron, however. Too much iron can be dangerous in large quantities, especially to men, who generally store more iron in their bodies than women do. Some studies have linked excessive iron to heart disease and cancer in men.

Folic Acid: A Good Pill for Certain Ills

Folic acid is responsible for the production of healthy red blood cells. When it's in short supply, anemia becomes likely. This type of anemia sometimes occurs in pregnant women, when the demand for folic acid is greater than the body's stores. Even if you aren't contemplating getting pregnant but are still in your childbearing years, you need to get enough folic acid every day. This B vitamin can be found in green leafy vegetables, organ meats, fortified foods, and many multivitamin tablets. Deficiencies in folic acid have been linked to spina bifida and anencephaly (the absence of a portion of the skull or brain) in infants. Supplementing your diet with folic acid can minimize the risk of these birth defects. But for folic acid to work, a sufficient quantity must be in your system during the early weeks of fetal development. If you wait until you know for sure you are pregnant, you may lose precious weeks.

Folic acid anemia can also occur in alcoholics, who may become malnourished if drinking is their major source of calories and their digestive tract ceases to absorb nutrients as well as it used to. This condition is treated through diet, folic acid supplementation, and a complete abstinence from alcohol.

Vitamin D: The Sunshine Vitamin

Vitamin D has recently received a great deal of attention from the research community. Studies show that taking between 400 and 600 international units of vitamin D daily appeared to reduce mortality rates from any cause. Other research shows a link between vitamin D deficiency and cancer, heart disease, and diabetes and an association between inadequate vitamin D intake and reduced muscle strength, higher risk of falls, and a decline in mental function.

Vitamin D is normally obtained in adequate amounts through a healthy diet. Some of the richest sources include wild salmon (3 ounces = 420 international units), Atlantic mackerel (3 ounces = 320 international units), sardines (1 can = 250 international units), shrimp (3 ounces = 150 international units), and shiitake mush-rooms (4 items = 260 international units). Other good sources are vitamin D–fortified dairy products and cereals.

You also absorb vitamin D through the skin with ten to twenty minutes of exposure daily. If you slather on a lot of sunscreen (still a good idea) or live in a rainier, cloudier clime, you're likely to be at a higher risk for a deficiency than those on whom the sun always shines. Should food and sun sources be in short supply, it's a good idea to consider supplements. Take a multivitamin which provides at least the daily value, 400 international units. For women taking extra calcium, buy a brand that also provides vitamin D. The most active—and best—form of vitamin D is D_3 (cholcalciferol).

Fish Oil for a Healthy Heart

Fish oil supplements are worth looking into if you have heart trouble. If you have elevated triglycerides, for example, the American Heart Association says you may need 2 to 4 grams of eicosapentaenoic acid (EPA) and docosahexaenoic acid (DHA) per day provided as capsules under a physician's care. If you have documented cardiovascular disease, the association recommends about 1 gram of EPA + DHA per day, preferably from fatty fish. Supplements are an option, too, but talk to your doctor about them. If you don't have heart disease, try to eat fatty fish at least two times a week. Examples of these types of fish include salmon, herring, and trout. Although many experts recommend fish oil supple-

TRUTH

Oysters deserve their aphrodisiac reputation.

Casanova is said to have braced himself with oysters before venturing into a lady's boudoir. Oysters (in fact, all seafood) are packed with minerals that are critical components of sex hormones. Minerals are also vital for optimal functioning of your brain and nervous system. One of these minerals is zinc, which has been associated with an increase in sperm motility, and theoretically increases a man's fertility. It also helps reduce the risk of inflammation of the prostate, a problem that can put a crimp in any man's love life.

ments, they admit that the oil inside the capsules may not be as effective as the naturally occurring oils in fish.

CALORIE RESTRICTION, AGING, AND SUPPLEMENTATION

Another group of people who need supplements are those who restrict calories as part of an antiaging lifestyle. While it has long been known that eating well and staying trim helps people live healthier lives as well as avoid dying prematurely, evidence has been accumulating that following extremely low-calorie diets (as low as 800 to 1,000 calories a day) for many years may do something more than keep you thin—it prolongs life.

The science is very persuasive. It seems that lab monkeys, rats, mice, and other critters live much longer when fed very low-calorie diets, and some researchers suggest the same fountain of youth effects hold true for us. Severe caloric restriction decreases circulating free radicals, harmful molecules in the body that age us. This decrease reduces oxidation, which is your body's version of rust on a car. With less oxidation, "telomeres" are less likely to shorten. Telomeres are the caps at the delicate ends of chromosomes, the molecules that carry genes. Every time a cell divides, telomeres shorten. As part of the normal aging process, telomeres eventually get so short that cells can no longer divide, and they die off. As more and more cells reach the end of their telomeres and die, the process produces the effects of aging. (Obesity causes telomeres to shorten, too, by the way—another incentive, if you're overweight, to try to knock off those extra pounds.)

One of the first human studies of calorie restriction showed calorie restrictors had younger hearts than normal-weight people on a typical Western diet. Other findings in people indicate that calorie restriction has a powerful protective effect against diseases associated with aging, such as heart attack, stroke, diabetes, and cancer.

Now for the downside (other than never being able to have the occasional potato chip or bowl of ice cream): If you're subsisting on 800 calories a day, you run the risk of malnutrition, so you have to turn to supplements. And I'm not talking about a vitamin or two. Many calorie-restriction disciples supplement with thirty, forty, or more pills a day.

Calorie restriction isn't practical for everyone—I sure couldn't do it—but its antiaging promise is appealing. Let's admit it—the prospect of dying meets with resistance in

TRUTH

"Natural" or "herbal" doesn't mean safe.

A product that claims to be "natural" or "herbal" is not necessarily safe. Tobacco is natural, for example, but we know it's a slow killer. So is arsenic. Also, some herbs and other natural therapies can interact with prescription and over-the-counter drugs. Women taking oral contraceptives should not take Saint-John's-wort, for example, because it can make birth control pills less effective. Vitamin E, garlic, ginkgo biloba, and a host of other herbs can increase bleeding and complications during surgery. Also, anyone taking the chemotherapy drug methotrexate should not supplement with folic acid. Tell your doctor or pharmacist about all supplements you are taking to avoid potentially dangerous nutrient-drug interactions.

all of us. But to live longer or eat that slice of cheesecake? I hope science finds a way to let us do both.

NATURAL WEIGHT-LOSS SUPPLEMENTS: BOGUS OR BENEFICIAL?

We've all watched, read, or listened to countless ads or infomercials selling a magic pill promising to solve all our diet struggles and give us the body we've always dreamed of having. It's not that easy. It takes a lot more than a bottle of pills to make you a real-life before-and-after photo.

And just because these dietary or weight-loss supplements claim to be made with herbs and other naturally occurring ingredients doesn't mean you can take them without worry. Dietary-supplement companies aren't required to show clinical data on their efficacy and safety to the FDA, which means we have no idea whether they work or if they're safe.

A good example is bitter orange extract, a substance that has replaced ephedra as an ingredient in many weight-loss supplements. Two products containing bitter orange increased blood pressure by 7 percent to 12 percent in participants in a University of California–San Francisco study. What's more, bitter orange doesn't appear to help people lose weight, according to a research review.

Another supplement that has received lots of hype but fails to help in the fat-burning department is carnitine. Its physiologic role in the body is to shuttle fat into the mitochondria (the energy centers of a cell) to be burned for energy. In theory, taking supplemental carnitine would enhance this fat-burning process. But this is just conjecture. Laboratory studies are inconclusive as to whether this actually works. Despite questionable find-

TRUTH

Sipping green tea may be slimming.

Green tea looks really interesting for weight loss. Studies suggest that beyond the caffeine in green tea (which boosts metabolism slightly), there appears to be a fat-burning effect from the tea itself. Drinking 4 to 6 cups of green tea per day seems to burn about 80 calories. That's quite a bit of tea and, in some people, could raise heart rate and blood pressure. But experts also say there have been no adverse effects reported from drinking green tea.

TRUTH

Apple cider vinegar may help with weight loss.

For thousands of years, vinegar has been used for weight loss, and no doubt you've heard of the apple cider vinegar diet. It turns out there might be some truth to this fad diet, after all. White vinegar (and perhaps other types) might help people feel full. A 2005 study found that those who ate a piece of bread along with small amounts of white vinegar felt fuller and more satisfied than those who just ate the bread. While the results of these studies are promising, we still don't know enough. More research is needed.

ings by scientists, some supplement manufacturers are still pushing the stuff as a legitimate fat burner.

And while there may be some truth to the weight-loss promises of hoodia, a spiny succulent said to be used by African Bushmen to stave off pain, hunger, and thirst during long-distance travel over the vast desert, a lot of the products that claim to be made with hoodia don't actually contain much or any at all. Whether hoodia itself is harmless is unknown, but products that use it often contain other questionable ingredients, such as bitter orange.

At last count, there were more than fifty individual dietary supplements and more than 125 commercial combination products available for weight loss. I've listed some of the more popular ingredients in the table that follows. Most are marketed on very flimsy evidence, and their safety and effectiveness are unclear. Many haven't even been studied in humans. Until more information is

TRUTH

Meal replacement products can help you lose weight.

Unlike the liquid protein diets of yesteryear or the stringent very low-calorie liquid fasts, the use of today's meal replacements in weight control not only works, according to a number of studies, but it also makes sense for busy lifestyles. Meal replacement products are not limited to shakes and bars, either. They now include prepackaged meals, like those from Lean Cuisine, Weight Watchers, Healthy Choice, and other food manufacturers that make calorie-controlled entrées.

The usual approach is to use a meal replacement for one or two meals a day while having sensible meals that combine lean meat, carbohydrate, vegetables, and fruit for the other meals during the day.

WHAT'S IN THAT NATURAL WEIGHT-LOSS FORMULA?

INGREDIENT	THE TRUTH
Bitter orange (citrus aurantium)	May be unsafe. Do not combine this supplement with decongestants, large amounts of caffeine, or other stimulants, as this could increase blood pressure and heart rate.
Conjugated linoleic acid (CLA)	CLA is a polyunsaturated, conjugated fatty acid that is found primarily in meat and dairy products. Most manufacturers convert linoleic acid from safflowers into CLA. Results of studies into fat loss have been mixed. None of the human studies have been long term.
Chromium	Most often present as chromium picolinate, this has been promoted to boost lean muscle mass and decrease body fat, though study findings have been generally inconclusive.
Green tea	Contains extracts that may increase metabolism.

INGREDIENT	THE TRUTH
Hoodia	A spiny succulent that grows in the desert. It contains a compound called P57 that tricks the body into thinking it's full. Preliminary research shows an appetite-suppressing benefit. A problem with hoodia is finding products that are pure and actually contain the active ingredient.
Hydroxycitric acid (HCA)	Promoted as an appetite suppressant, although unproven, HCA may cause nausea, GI discomfort, and/or headache.
7-Keto DHEA	Don't confuse this with the hormone DHEA. 7-Keto DHEA claims to increase metabolism; one small study showed that it reversed the decrease in RMR normally associated with dieting, but the study was too small to be conclusive.
Phaseolamin vulgaris	Extracted from the white kidney bean, this ingredient supposedly works by allowing carbohydrates to pass through the gastrointestinal system undigested. Studies also show it can decrease the absorption of glucose from a full meal.
Pyruvate	Pyruvate supplements boast that they stimulate metabolism and reduce body fat. Pyruvate is found naturally in food and in the body as a result of the breakdown of carbohydrates and protein. Some studies have shown a weight-loss benefit, but the people in the studies also exercised and cut back on calories. Moreover, the dosage used in the studies was high, requiring a handful of tablets each day. Large doses (5 grams or more daily) may lead to abdominal bloating, gas, and/or diarrhea. Experts say the case for pyruvate as an aid to weight loss is weak.
Stimulant herbs	Although it may not be listed on a label, several metabolism-boosting herbs naturally contain caffeine, such as green and black tea, guarana, kola nut, cacao, and yerba mate. Any caffeine-containing substance can disrupt sleep, particularly if taken later in the day or in high doses.

known, I cannot endorse natural products for weight loss. Ten years from now, I may be singing a different tune—but not yet.

SIDE EFFECTS OF VITAMIN MEGADOSES

VITAMIN	DRI/UL*	SIDE EFFECTS FROM MEGADOSING
Vitamin A (retinol, retinal, retinoic acid)	**DRI:** Women, 2,310 IU; pregnant women, 2,565 IU; lactating women, 4,300 IU; men, 3,000 IU **UL:** 10,000 IU (adults)	Nausea Vomiting Headache Dizziness Blurred vision Clumsiness Birth defects Liver problems Possible risk of osteoporosis (You may be at greater risk of these effects if you drink high amounts of alcohol, have liver problems, have high cholesterol levels, or don't get enough protein.)
Vitamin D (calciferol)	**DRI:** Women, ages 19–50, 200 IU; women, ages 51–70, 400 IU; women age 70+, 600 IU; men, ages 19–50, 200 IU; men, ages 51–70, 400 IU; men age 70+, 600 IU **UL:** 2,000 IU (adults)	Nausea Vomiting Poor appetite Constipation Weakness Weight loss Confusion Heart rhythm problems Deposits of calcium and phosphate in soft tissues
Vitamin E	**DRI:** 15 mg; lactating women, 19 mg; doctors advise against taking more than 400 mg a day (although the UL is 1,000 mg)	Dangerous thinning of the blood
Vitamin K	**DRI:** Women, 90 micrograms (mcg); men, 120 mcg **UL:** Not established	Dangerous thinning of the blood

VITAMIN	DRI/UL*	SIDE EFFECTS FROM MEGADOSING
Vitamin B$_3$ (niacin)	**DRI:** Women, 14 mg; pregnant women, 18 mg; lactating women, 17 mg; men, 16 mg **UL:** 35 mg	Flushing Redness of the skin Upset stomach
Vitamin B$_6$ (pyridoxine, pyridoxal, and pyridoxamine)	**DRI:** Women, ages 9–30, 1.3 mg; women ages 31–70, 1.5 mg; pregnant women, 1.9 mg; lactating women, 2.0 mg; men, ages 19–30, 1.3 mg; men ages 31–70, 1.7 mg **UL:** 100 mcg	Nerve damage to the limbs, which may cause numbness Trouble walking
Vitamin C	**DRI:** Women, 75 mg; pregnant women, 85 mg; lactating women, 120 mg; men, 90 mg; also: 110 mg for female smokers and 130 mg for male smokers **UL:** 2,000 mg	Upset stomach Kidney stones Increased iron absorption
Folic acid (folate)	**DRI:** Women, 400 mcg; pregnant women, 600 mcg; lactating women, 500 mcg; men, 400 mcg **UL:** 1,000 mcg	High levels may, especially in older adults, hide signs of B$_{12}$ deficiency, a condition that can cause nerve damage

DRI, or daily reference intake, is a method of rating the amount of a nutrient we need for good health. UL refers to tolerable upper intake levels that apply to healthy people. ULs represent the maximum intake of a nutrient that is likely to pose no health risks. Taking more than the UL is not recommended and may be harmful.

As for supplements in general, we shouldn't be putting anything in our mouths until we know whether it works. The truth comes to light when you look at the science. Remember, if it sounds too good to be true, it usually is.

Myth #9

Low-Fat Diets Are a Waste of Time

The year was 1988. The place was San Francisco. I had moved to California's fourth-most populous city that year to find a new life. I had lined up two jobs, one with the University of California–San Francisco, the other with a local television station. Those of you who have heard me speak or who have read my books know I'm open to a variety of approaches that fall outside mainstream medicine. When I heard that a controversial young internist, who said he could reverse heart disease naturally, was going to speak at a medical meeting in my newly adopted town, I grabbed my notepad and pen, and off I went to hear what he had to say.

The tall, lean, wiry-haired physician began his lecture by showing us a slide of doctors busily mopping up a wet floor around a sink that is overflowing, with no one turning off the faucet. In that metaphor was a powerful, eye-opening message: We doctors treat the symptoms of disease without ever treating the cause. He went on to say, "If you treat the cause, you turn off the faucet, which for many people represents their diet and lifestyle choices, so the need for medication and the need for surgery are often greatly reduced."

The next few slides showed the really ugly blocked and diseased arteries of one of his patients. The next slide revealed something quite remarkable: the same person's arteries but smoother and more open. What had produced these near-miraculous changes? An intensive multimonth course of a low-fat diet (10 percent of daily calories came from fat), regular exercise, stress-reducing meditation, and, of course, no smoking. His point? Heart disease is reversible.

The young internist, of course, was Dr. Dean Ornish. The now internationally recognized physician has become known for his lifestyle-oriented, no-nonsense approach to avoiding bypass surgery and maintaining cardiovascular health. His dietary prescription is not just vegetarian. It also has little or no added salt, fat, or oil. He allows virtually no sugar.

Ornish is an adherent of his own program. In 1972 he dropped out of Rice University in Houston to recover from mononucleosis and depression. At his parents' home in Dallas, Dr. Ornish met a swami, who had been guiding Dr. Ornish's older sister in meditation and relaxation techniques. Dr. Ornish asked the swami to help him, too—which entailed becoming a vegetarian, practicing yoga, meditating, and helping others. Dr. Ornish felt better and more peaceful. The swami virtually handed him what would become the Ornish program.

Although impressed with the advancements of coronary bypass surgery that were part of his medical training, Dr. Ornish was troubled by the fact that patients were sent home, thinking they were cured, only to resume the unhealthy habits that brought them to the hospital in the first place. They continued to smoke, eat a diet high in saturated fat, lead stressful lives, and avoid regular exercise. The young medical student reasoned that if you addressed the causes of heart disease, patients could avoid costly, and possibly dangerous, surgery and save their lives.

Dr. Ornish was eager to see whether the program he learned from the swami would reverse heart disease. He gathered up ten patients. Half chose to follow his program; the others did not. He taught them nutrition and yoga. He led them in a support group where they could share their troubles. Those who followed his program ended up with lower blood levels of cholesterol, less chest pain, and improved heart function. He followed this study with a yearlong study of forty-eight volunteers with severe heart disease. Half of the group began Dr. Ornish's rigorous regimen, while half followed less stringent conventional recommendations, which advised only modest dietary changes, light exercise, and quitting smoking.

The results were dramatic. Those on Dr. Ornish's regimen began to feel better quickly. They experienced a dramatic drop in cholesterol levels, weight, and angina (chest pain). Angiograms showed that blocked arteries in the participants had begun to clear. In frightening contrast, the majority of those in the control group became measurably worse during the same interval.

Other exciting discoveries followed. Dr. Ornish had assumed that only younger patients with milder disease would be likely to show reversal, but he was wrong, thankfully. Improvement wasn't based on how old or sick someone was. It was based on how much they changed their diet and lifestyle—in other words, how closely they stuck to his program. In fact, he found the greatest degree of reversal in an eighty-three-year-old man! Many patients under their doctor's supervision have been able to reduce and, in some cases, get off of medications completely, when they follow Dr. Ornish's program.

To this day, Dr. Ornish believes that the American Heart Association's recommendation to pare fat down to only 30 percent of your daily calories is too liberal. His beliefs are bold, and many in the medical establishment consider him a renegade. But he continues to stand his ground: heart disease can be reversed with the help of a low-fat diet and other lifestyle changes.

After hearing what he had to say back in 1988, I decided to try his low-fat diet for myself. Dean was gracious enough to have the same meals that his patients were eating delivered to my house. For three weeks, I ate a rigid low-fat diet, and I didn't cheat. (But I sure wanted to!) It was tough but it worked. I felt better and I lost nearly 8 pounds.

It was a departure, though, from my idea of moderation, and a diet that, in the absence of heart disease, I could not continue for months on end.

In our society, we eat too much fat and too little fiber,

and we lead lives that are too sedentary. It wasn't always that way. It happened over the past few decades, and now we are paying the price. Dr. Ornish's patients are living testaments to the fact that what you put in your mouth has a direct effect on your heart and on your body. A low-fat diet certainly has its place at the health table.

ANATOMY OF A MYTH

Ever feel like throwing up your hands as you slog through nutritional information about fats? Fats used to be simple to understand. Butter is bad. Margarine is good. Vegetable oils are healthy. And too much fat of any kind is harmful for you. But these easy guidelines gave way to a perplexing—and at times contradictory—buffet of dietary do's and don'ts. Salads with a little olive oil are okay. Candies made with coconut oil aren't. Fish oil gets a green light. Margarine is verboten. Butter is back.

In the early 1990s all fats were bad and all carbs were good. Americans went on low-fat diets, renouncing fat for carbs in the name of better health. Everybody filled up on foods loaded with added sugars and refined starches that had little to offer nutritionally besides calories. They assumed that if a food had no fat, they could eat as much of it as they wanted, not realizing that many low-fat and fat-free products have nearly as many calories as their full-fat versions. And so, Americans grew fatter.

Then came a backlash. Instead of low-fat diets, some researchers said, we should be emphasizing low-carbohydrate diets, the very opposite of what we had been told.

To make matters worse for fats, along came an anti-low-fat diet dispatch published in the *Journal of the American Medical Association* in 2006. A massive, federally funded study, part of a much larger project called the Women's Health Initiative, proclaimed that low-fat diets—long recommended as the path to better health—don't help much. The study of nearly fifty thousand postmenopausal women (average age sixty-two) found that eating low-fat diets for eight years offered no health benefits—no lowered risk for heart disease, colon cancer, or breast cancer. The results confounded conventional wisdom and standard medical advice.

But as is often the case, the diet news was misinterpreted, and you had to read between the lines. True, after an average of eight years, researchers found no statistically significant difference in breast cancer risk between women on a low-fat diet and women who had made no changes in what they ate. But that's not the bottom line. The women who had the highest fat consumption at the start of the trial and who managed to cut it back the closest to 20 percent for the longest period developed 22 percent fewer breast cancers than the women in the control group. That is significant. Scientists will observe the women until 2010, so stay tuned for a whole new message about the value of low-fat eating.

Furthermore, the women in the intervention group had 9 percent fewer polyps and other precancerous growths in their lower gastrointestinal tract. Given that it takes a decade or more for colorectal cancer to develop, it may be too soon to see if there's a corresponding drop in cancer rates. As for heart disease, the investigators tracked only the total amount of fat consumed and not the saturated and trans fats (both are "bad fats") now known to damage arteries.

Even so, these have not been good times for low-fat diets.

But are they a waste of time and effort?

No, this is a huge myth that has been gathering steam for decades. There is too much other evidence that reducing your fat intake, particularly from certain types of "bad fats," will indeed lower your risk of heart disease, stroke, cancer, and other diseases. We should all lower our fat intake (I'll give you recommendations), exercise regularly, and eat more fruits, vegetables, and fiber-rich whole grains.

TRUTH

You don't need to give up dessert to lose weight.

Try these strategies: Reduce the serving sizes of your meal to save calorie room for dessert. Cut back on the amount of dessert. For example, instead of two scoops of ice cream, have one. Or share a dessert with a friend. Make desserts more nutritious. For example, use whole grains, fresh fruit, and applesauce when preparing desserts. Many times, you can use less sugar and fat than a recipe calls for without sacrificing taste or texture.

LOW-FAT DIETS AND WEIGHT LOSS

Over the years, a spate of studies comparing low-carb versus low-fat diets has confirmed that, generally, both diets take weight off because both restrict calories. A higher-fat diet is appealing, but I'm afraid that if people believe they can eat more fat calories, they will eat fewer plant foods, get fewer natural antioxidants, and not consume enough fiber—bad habits that are already a part of our profile. And we don't have a prayer of dealing with the growing obesity problem in this country if we say there's nothing wrong with eating fat, because gram for gram, fat contains more calories than either carbs or protein. Cutting back on fats just makes sense if you're trying to slim down.

Remember, weight gain is not about carbs or fat per se. It's about calories. Eat fewer calories than you burn off, and you'll lose weight. And you don't have to adopt a trendy diet to do that. The only distinction that counts is the one between nutritious food and junk. Give up refined carbs—foods made with white sugar and flour, ranging from sodas to sugary breakfast cereals—and you'll automatically control your calories. These processed foods fail to fill you up until you've eaten way too many calories, and they contain little to no nutritional value. And they're absorbed quickly into the bloodstream, prompting the body to unleash a surge of insulin that accelerates the conversion of calories into fat.

By contrast, fruits, vegetables, and whole grains are densely packed with life-sustaining compounds. They're absorbed gradually enough to prevent sudden insulin spikes. And they satisfy better, thanks to their high fiber and fluid content. Eat an apple, and you have a filling, healthful snack for 80 calories. Plow through even a few cookies and before you know it you've inhaled 600 empty calories.

Giving up junk food is easier than you might think. Whole, fresh food offers sensual delights that fast food could never match. If you think about it, it's junk food that's tasteless, requiring large amounts of salt, corn syrup, and trans fats to make it palatable. If you forget about the war between fats and carbs and focus instead on nutritional value, you'll have a diet that is not only healthier but more delicious.

For more than thirty years, I've been telling my patients, friends, family, viewers, anyone who would listen,

TRUTH

Diets do work.

The phrase *diets don't work* has been drummed into us by book titles, advertising slogans, and other such mantras. But the truth is, you can lose weight following pretty much every diet on the bookstore shelf. The problem is that unless the diet fits your lifestyle, it's bound to fail, and your weight will creep back on. You want a diet you can live with.

If you like sandwiches for lunch, for example, you'll have trouble sticking to a low-carb diet. If you hate counting calories and find it much easier to follow rules—like avoiding carbs—Atkins may be for you. And if you really love your olive oil, the Mediterranean diet is more appealing than a true low-fat diet. If you're trying to lose weight, you have to exercise your options.

how to eat a healthful diet. Don't scrimp on fruits, vegetables, or whole grains. Pick lean sources of protein. Limit your fat intake to around 20 percent of your total daily calories. Stay active. Those who follow this advice will lose weight—and keep it off.

LOW-FAT DIETS KEEP YOU LEAN FOR LIFE

Here's the best news about low-fat diets: Dieters who want to keep from regaining the pounds they so painstakingly lost would do best to follow a low-fat diet rather than curb carbs.

The proof is found in the University of Colorado–based National Weight Control Registry, which tracks dieters who have kept off 30 pounds or more for at least a year. What's their secret? They eat a low-fat diet and watch their total calories. And they get sixty to ninety minutes of exercise a day.

One study from the registry found that people reported eating about 1,400 calories a day, with the portion that came from fat at about 29 percent and about 50 percent from carbs. Those who increased their fat intake after their initial weight loss regained the most weight. Only a minority of long-term weight losers were following low-carbohydrate diets.

It probably doesn't matter much what kind of diet you follow to lose weight initially, but keeping from regaining it is another matter altogether. Study after study shows that a low-fat diet continues to be a key element to long-term success.

TRUTH

Fast foods can be a healthy choice for dieters.

These days, fast-food companies publish the nutrient information, including calories, for all their menu items. A little calorie know-how can thus help you make healthy choices. For example, choose salads (dressing on the side) and grilled foods over fried foods. At the same time, don't deprive yourself. Enjoy higher-calorie items as a treat (my Treat Yourself Diet gives you that option), or have them in smaller portions.

RESURRECTING THE LOW-FAT DIET

There's no real definition of a low-fat diet, but to most people it generally means a food plan in which 20 to 30 percent of your total calories comes from fat, with an emphasis on whole grains, fruits, vegetables, and other foods that fill you up without supplying many calories. But to others, a low-fat diet doesn't mean cantaloupe and carrot sticks. It's an invitation to an all-you-can-eat buffet of high-calorie foods like fat-free cakes, cookies, ice cream, and chips. That's not healthy dieting; that's a dieting disaster.

If you're convinced that it might not be a bad idea to monitor the fat in your diet, I'll give you two ways of doing it, first, the "real" formula and then the "easy" way.

The formula really isn't that tricky. Figure out how many calories you need to eat in a day (see page 66). As an example, let's use 1,500 calories. Multiply that number by 0.2, since 20 percent of your calories should come from fat. Then divide that number by 9, since there are 9 calories in each gram of fat. That will give you the total number of fat grams you should eat in one day.

So it works like this:

$$1{,}500 \text{ calories} \times 0.2 = 300$$
$$300 \div 9 = 33$$

You should eat no more than 33 grams of fat per day.

The easy way is to play down the numbers, forget the math, and focus instead on plain old foods—fruits, vegetables, legumes, whole grains, and fish—that will help most Americans prevent heart disease, hypertension, and stroke. If you follow this advice, your dietary percentages will fall into line naturally. In effect, your plate will do the math for you. There won't be much room to add lots of extra oil, and you'll automatically reduce fat. Enough good fat will creep into your diet, anyway.

TRUTH

Blotting your pizza will cut down on some fat and calories.

While it won't soak up all of the fat and calories, it can make a dent. If you're eating a medium slice of cheese pizza, swabbing it first with a napkin can remove up to 45 calories and 5 grams of fat. But all the mopping in the world won't help if you're ordering the wrong kind of pizza. Some pizzas, namely, the stuffed-crust and meat-lovers varieties, can clock in at 800 calories per slice and contain more than a day's worth of fat and sodium. Also, switching from deep dish to thin crust can also slash up to 200 calories and 6 grams of fat.

ALL FATS ARE NOT CREATED EQUAL

We need a little fat in our diets for good health, and some fats are better for you than others. Fatty acids, the building blocks for fat, are divided into three chemical classes according to their hydrogen content: saturated, monounsaturated, and polyunsaturated. Here's a rundown.

Saturated Fatty Acids

Saturated fats are the main culprit in raising low-density lipoproteins (LDL, or "bad" cholesterol). They are found primarily in meats and dairy products. Many of these foods also contain cholesterol. Cutting down on saturated fat means going easy on beef, veal, lamb, pork, beef and poultry fat, butter, cream, whole milk, and cheeses as well as other dairy products made from whole milk. Saturated fatty acids are also found in plant-based products, including palm and coconut oils and cocoa butter. The

TRUTH

There's no need to shun red meat on a low-fat diet.

While it's true that prime and choice grades of meat are high in fat, lean cuts with fewer than 30 percent calories as fat are available. When buying meat, it's best to look for "select" grades of lean cuts like top round and tenderloin as well as extra-lean ground beef. They are among the lowest in fat.

American Heart Association recommends that you limit your saturated fat intake to less than 10 percent of total calories each day. The less the better. This is a "bad" fat.

Polyunsaturated Fats

These are typically found in the liquid oils that come from vegetables. Common sources include sesame, sunflower, and safflower oils; sunflower seeds; and corn and soybeans and their oils. Only the polyunsaturated fats are considered "essential," meaning they cannot be manufactured by the body. Like minerals and vitamins, they must be ingested as food. If we don't eat enough, then we won't get enough. And that would be unfortunate, for these compounds—principally linoleic acid and linolenic acid—are vital to the maintenance of cell membranes and to the manufacture of potent chemical messengers that regulate everything from blood pressure to the firing of nerves.

When essential fatty acids are in short supply, the body compensates by substituting other types of fatty acids that have a less supple biochemical structure. As polyunsaturates are replaced by these other compounds, cell membranes become more rigid, leading to progressive hardening of the arterial walls. Polyunsaturated fats should make up 10 percent or less of your total daily calories. They are "good" fats.

I should also emphasize another type of essential polyunsaturated fat: omega-3 fatty acids. These are found in fatty fish, like salmon, tuna, and trout, as well as in

TRUTH

Elevated levels of mercury have been found in large, long-living ocean fish.

These include shark, swordfish, king mackerel, tilefish, and halibut—as well as freshwater fish living in contaminated waters. Exposure to high mercury levels can affect neurological development, which is why some experts advise that women of childbearing age, pregnant and nursing women, and children younger than age eight avoid large ocean fish and be extremely cautious about other fish. Eating up to 12 ounces per week of a variety of smaller ocean fish, shellfish, or farm-raised fish should be fine for women. And it's prudent to minimize the amount of white canned tuna your family consumes. Limit a child to 4 ounces of store-bought tuna or 2 ounces of freshly caught cooked fish per week. Also check with your local and state health department or environmental agency to make sure your local waters are clean before you eat any fish you catch.

canola oil and flaxseed. Known as eicosapentaenoic acid, or EPA, and docosahexaenoic acid, or DHA, they help maintain and protect your heart, blood vessels, and brain function. Two fish meals a week will supply you with the right amount of these fats.

Monounsaturated Fatty Acids

Monounsaturated fats come from avocados and olive, canola, and peanut oils, as well as from nuts. For more than thirty-five years, studies have shown that diets containing monounsaturated fats, such as the traditional Mediterranean diet, are good for the heart. These fats can help lower cholesterol, blood pressure, and blood

TRUTH

Pork is one of the leanest sources of protein.

If it's pork tenderloin, that is. With just 122 calories per 3 ounces, pork tenderloin is very lean, supplying as much protein as prime rib for one-third to one-eighth of the fat. The same size serving of pork top loin has 147 calories and 5 grams of fat.

sugar levels. The Mediterranean diet is moderately high in fat (about 30 percent of fat calories mostly from olive oil) and emphasizes fresh fruits and vegetables, whole grains, legumes, nuts, and a high intake of fish and little red meat. If your HDL (high-density lipoprotein, or "good") cholesterol is low (35 or less), add a daily serving or two of canola or olive oil, nuts, avocado, or fatty fish (like salmon). In exchange, subtract a serving or two of sweets or refined bread, pasta, crackers, or cereal.

These "good" fats should make up about 15 percent of your total calories. Both polyunsaturated and monounsaturated fats are better than saturated fats because they may aid in lowering cholesterol. But remember they are fats and should still be used sparingly. They are not a license to add oil; their calories do count.

Trans Fats

One type of bad fat to eliminate entirely is trans fat, also known as partially hydrogenated vegetable oil. Trans fats are formed during a process called hydrogenation, which

TRUTH

When you blow your diet, get back on track with your next meal.

When they fall off the diet wagon, most people wait until the next day to restart their diet. That racks up even more calories—and possibly more pounds. Every meal counts, so if you ate that big old piece of birthday cake at lunch, get right back on track at dinner.

transforms liquid oil into shelf-stable solid fat. Trans fats clog arteries, and are found in many packaged cookies, crackers, snacks, and other processed foods.

READ LABELS

Be aware, too, that fat is hiding everywhere—in places where you would least expect it, so you have to be a smart label reader. Look at the number of grams of fat (the lower the better) and figure it into your daily allotment.

Also note how much saturated fat makes up the total because this is the fat that clogs arteries. It is always listed separately because it's a risky element. That number should be less than 30 percent. Figuring out the percentage can be a little tricky, so I always fall back on trying to limit the total number of fat grams. It's faster and easier.

Finally, search for cholesterol. The American Heart

TRUTH

Food products labeled "no cholesterol" aren't necessarily heart healthy.

The "no cholesterol" label doesn't mean that an item is fat-free. The key to watch for is the cholesterol and fat content of foods. Avoid fried foods. Cook with unsaturated vegetable oils instead of butter, or use applesauce or fruit puree in place of all or part of the oil in desserts. Substitute skim-milk products for whole-milk counterparts. When recipes call for eggs, replace one egg with two egg whites to cut out some cholesterol.

Association calls cholesterol "a second cousin to fat." Again, the lower the better, since too much cholesterol can raise the risk of heart disease. The American Heart Association recommends eating less than 300 milligrams of cholesterol a day.

TRUTH

The less fat you eat, the less fat you'll want.

Your desire for the taste of fat can vanish. A follow-up study of participants in the Women's Health Trial found that those eating a diet of only 20 percent fat developed aversions to the high-fat foods they used to prefer. So try skim and low-fat dairy products, and when baking substitute fruit purees for fats and evaporated skim milk for heavy cream in recipes. It takes a few weeks, but you really can retrain your tastes to prefer the lighter versions.

FIVE GREAT MEDICAL REASONS TO CONSIDER A LOW-FAT DIET

Experts can debate the pros and cons of monos and polys versus carbs until the carrots come home. You need to know what to eat today. The optimal diet for good health depends on who you are as well as what you want to achieve. I have suggestions that may help you decide whether a low-fat diet is right for you.

You Want to Prevent Heart Disease

The best place to begin is reducing the saturated fat and the trans fat in your diet. Numerous studies show that saturated fat increases inflammation, raises cholesterol, and leads to the accumulation of fatty plaques inside blood vessel walls (atherosclerosis). Those plaques can rupture, form artery-blocking blood clots, and lead to a heart attack. Saturated fat is also associated with stroke and obesity.

Trans fats are even worse. In addition to raising "bad" LDL cholesterol, they lower "good" HDL cholesterol—something saturated fat doesn't do. Other research has linked trans fats to Alzheimer's disease, age-related macular degeneration, and inflammation (also linked to cancer).

You've Been Diagnosed with Heart Disease

I limit the amount of fat in my own diet, especially since a computed tomography scan of my heart a few years ago revealed some unfriendly plaque. To say I was surprised and upset would be an understatement. I've never smoked. I'm not overweight, and my BMI is normal. I'm not genetically inclined toward heart disease. This was unthinkable and nearly impossible to absorb. Heart disease doesn't just spring up overnight out of nowhere, however. Through a thousand flashbacks, I remembered how I ate in college and medical school, and the big picture suddenly made sense. All those years of subsisting on fatty burgers and french fries, and now I'm paying for the nutritional sins of my youth.

A low-fat diet can be helpful for treating heart disease. You might want to consider Dr. Ornish's diet. He suggests that if you stick with a nonfat vegetarian diet, enough fat will slip in anyway to take care of bodily needs, and at the same time you'll be improving your heart health. So, if you already have cardiovascular disease, extremely low-fat diets can help unclog arteries.

For some people, Dr. Ornish's suggestions may be too hard to follow. As I said, I tried it, but for me the best route is somewhere in the middle. I try to eat no more than 20 grams of fat a day. I waved good-bye to fatty meats, resolved to get more exercise, and embraced vegetables as a formal religion. I am also taking a cholesterol-lowering drug, joining the ranks of millions of Americans who are on statins. Doing all of this, I expect my heart condition to reverse itself.

You Have High Blood Pressure

I'm extremely lucky: On any given day, my blood pressure hovers around 90 over 70—a reading doctors consider optimal. Normal pressure is actually 129 over 84 or below. Unfortunately, right now about fifty million Americans have high blood pressure, otherwise known as hypertension, defined as 140 over 90 or above.

Most of us never think about our blood pressure because we can't feel it. High blood pressure, in fact, is often a silent stalker. The longer it goes undiagnosed and untreated, the greater the risk for heart disease, stroke, or kidney problems.

Some people are genetically predisposed to high blood pressure. As for the rest of us, growing older, being overweight or inactive, or smoking can cause arteries to stiffen, making it difficult for blood to pass through.

Fortunately, most people can stave off high blood pressure by making simple lifestyle changes, such as exercising and following a low-fat diet. The Dietary Approaches to Stop Hypertension (DASH) diet has been shown in studies to help lower blood pressure and cholesterol. It has other benefits, too: An analysis of 88,517 women in the ongoing Nurses' Health Study showed that the diet also reduces the risk of developing coronary heart disease by 24 percent and stroke by 18 percent. The DASH diet, developed in the 1990s by researchers at the National Heart, Lung, and Blood Institute, is low in cholesterol and sodium, and contains no more than 30 percent of its calories from fat. It emphasizes fruits, vegetables, and fat-free or low-fat dairy products.

Have your blood pressure checked at least once every two years. If it's higher than normal, your doctor should repeatedly check it at several follow-up visits. It's up to your health-care provider to tell you when your blood pressure is creeping up and to prescribe treatment.

You Want to Prevent Breast Cancer, or Its Recurrence

Ask your gynecologist about the best ways to prevent breast cancer, and you're likely to hear about a number of things you can't easily control: being born with the right genes, hitting puberty later than age twelve, and having your first child before you're thirty. Those are not exactly a basis for action. Increasingly, though, physicians are mentioning a few things you can do that just might help reduce the frightening one-in-eight odds of getting breast cancer. They include keeping to a low-fat diet, watching your weight, avoiding stress, and getting plenty of exercise.

Cutting back on fat does, however, make sense in theory. Between 60 percent and 70 percent of primary breast cancers are hormone dependent, meaning they grow in response to estrogen. Excess dietary fat primes the ovaries to release more estrogen, which in turn promotes tumor growth.

Of course, the type of fat might make a difference when it comes to breast cancer. One report in the *Journal of the National Cancer Institute* found that women who consumed olive oil at more than one meal daily have a 25 percent lower risk of breast cancer than those who ingest it once a day or less. The study also found protective effects from a high consumption of fruits and vegetables. These findings reinforce the belief of some scientists that

TRUTH

Coffee revs up your metabolism.

Java can stoke your calorie-burning furnace, provided you drink it black. A study in the journal *Metabolism* found that the caffeine in 2 cups of coffee may cause a 145-pound woman to expend up to 50 extra calories over the next four hours. Caffeine stimulates your nervous system, signaling the body to release a small amount of energy from its fat stores. Stirring in milk, cream, or sugar, however, can cause your insulin levels to rise, which diminishes that metabolic effect.

Coffee is not for everyone, since it contains caffeine. Avoid caffeine if you suffer from restlessness, anxiety, irritability and/or headaches, or sleep problems; gastrointestinal problems; irritable bowel syndrome or ulcers; elevated blood pressure or abnormal heart rhythms; or premenstrual syndrome or fibrocystic breasts.

the traditional Mediterranean diet is healthier than the average American diet. Even so, studies don't consistently show that low-fat diets lead to less cancer. That may be because other dietary elements, including overall calories, also influence tumor development by affecting growth factors and hormones like insulin, which also promote cancer.

The strongest evidence that lifestyle may make a difference comes from studies of women who have already had breast cancer. A study from the National Cancer Institute found that in postmenopausal women who had had breast cancer, lowering fat intake to about 33 grams a day (about 20 percent of total calories) reduced the odds of a recurrence by 20 percent. This is not a huge gain, but if you are one of those who benefit from the reduced

TRUTH

Food combining doesn't help you lose weight.

Food combining is the practice of eating carbs, fat, and protein at separate meals to lose weight. The theory is that different food types (proteins, fats, starches, sugars, and acidic foods) require their own digestive enzymes to be metabolized properly. Some claim that mixing these groups or eating them at the wrong times could cause digestive issues or weight gain. For advocates of this eating style, having orange juice and scrambled eggs at a sitting, or even a turkey sandwich, is forbidden.

There is no proven benefit to food combining.

odds, it's well worth the effort. If you've been treated for breast cancer, switching to a low-fat diet makes sense. A dietitian can help get you started.

You Want to Reduce Your Risk of Alzheimer's Disease

Alzheimer's disease is caused by a disintegration of brain cells and is considered a form of dementia. There is a lot of controversy about whether it can be prevented with lifestyle changes, since the disease has a genetic component. More research is shedding light on this issue, and one bright spot is that eating plenty of fruits and vegetables, fish, and omega-3 rich oils—and less saturated fat and trans fats—may decrease the risk of dementia and Alzheimer's disease. You just can't go wrong by switching to a predominantly vegetable-based diet, with healthy fats included in your daily allotment of calories.

Trim the Harmful Fats in Your Diet and Include More of the Good Ones

- Buy skim milk for drinking and use it in recipes.
- Use full-fat cheese sparingly; look for cheese labeled "low fat" or buy mozzarella or ricotta, both of which are lower in fat.
- Make smart low-fat substitutions: mustard for mayonnaise; applesauce for oil in baking; two egg whites instead of a whole egg in recipes; and chilled, whipped evaporated milk for whipped cream.
- Switch to low-fat or nonfat dairy foods; for example, substitute yogurt for sour cream.
- Buy meats labeled "extra lean," such as lean ground beef or turkey.
- Trim the fat from meat and remove chicken skin before cooking, or purchase skinless poultry.
- Eat fish twice a week, especially those high in omega-3 fats.
- Go vegetarian a couple of days a week, substituting beans or legumes for a main dish.
- Make your own salad dressing with olive or canola oil. Try lemon juice with a dash of olive oil, or use balsamic vinegar for vinaigrette dressings.
- Make sure to buy products labeled "trans free."
- Broil or bake instead of frying; use vegetable cooking oil sprays for sautéing.
- Include nuts in your diet; snack on a handful of nuts instead of chips.

As for the fat debate, you could get awfully hungry waiting for scientists to come to a consensus. In the meantime, the next time someone asks you, "Hey, wasn't there a study that proved that low-fat diets aren't worth it?" you can just smile and ask that person to pass the peas.

EXTRA, EXTRA

Good fats help you feel full.

Nothing sabotages a diet like hunger. Let's face it, it's much easier to stay on track with a healthy eating plan when you're feeling full (or at the very least not hungry). Scientists have a name for this feeling: satiety.

To lose weight, we have to eat less (particularly of the wrong foods, which often produce cravings of their own). When we eat less, however, we may feel hungry, and most of us cannot resist hunger very long. That's why the average weight-loss diet lasts less than three weeks. But if you're not hungry, it's easier to stick with your eating plan.

Enter olive oil and other healthy unsaturated fats. They contain a fatty acid that helps keep the body satisfied and makes it possible to prolong the time between meals. Consuming a small amount of foods rich in these oils activates an appetite control switch in the brain. Because these oils are so effective in turning off your appetite, you only need a small amount (less than a tablespoon). To keep your appetite under control, have a little olive oil on your salad.

Myth #10

You Can't Keep Weight Off

I searched for Laura among a throng of people inside our local coffee shop. I was late, running behind from dropping my son off at school. I wove in and out of the crowd like a pond skater but couldn't find Laura. A hand shot up several heads in front of me. "Nancy!" The voice was hers. Had it not been for her wide-spaced green eyes and freckly complexion, I would not have recognized her. Laura, age fifty-eight, used to be quite heavy but was now lean and healthy looking in size 6 jeans and a red boat-necked sweater.

We hugged and exchanged the usual pleasantries about the brisk fall weather and how hard it is to find a parking place in downtown Princeton on Saturdays, and I apologized for being late. As two women usually do, we chimed, practically in chorus, "You look great!" Kvetching together about our appearance (or flaws) is always a bonding experience for women. And of course, Laura really did look great—a good 30 or 40 pounds trimmer since I had last seen her.

I first met Laura about nine years ago when I worked for Johnson & Johnson. Since then, she had retired and moved west and was back in town for a visit. Naturally, our conversation wended around to her spectacular weight loss.

Laura had been a little heavy in childhood. But like mine, her weight odyssey really began in college when she gained the "freshman 15" and then continued upward after she got married and had three children. "Before I knew it, I'd gotten up to 176 pounds, and I'm just five foot three," she said. Laura, an admitted "emotional eater," hovered at that weight for years.

I asked her what had spurred her to lose weight.

"Something unstoppable was coming over me. I was becoming my mother," Laura said in a loving tone, and bowed her head.

Laura's mother, who had also battled a weight problem, had died of breast cancer seven years ago. It was a tragic yet transforming time for Laura. She was afraid that her weight would increase her own risk. "It was a real wake-up call," she said.

Breast cancer is a very complicated illness. We do not know its cause, and there is likely more than one culprit. Weight may be a factor, however. Prior to menopause, women who are overweight may enjoy a slightly reduced risk of breast cancer, most likely because they ovulate less often than do slimmer women, so their breasts are exposed to less estrogen. Estrogen fuels the growth of breast cancer cells. After menopause, however, heavier women are at greater risk. That's probably because once the ovaries stop churning out estrogen, the body's fat cells become its primary source of the hormone. Losing excess weight is one concrete step that women can take to reduce the risk of developing breast cancer after menopause. That's what Laura did.

"I thought hard about myself and decided to make some changes," she explained. "I was scared, but I was also tired of being unhappy with my weight and not doing anything about it. So I started jogging a little bit. After a month, the jogging became running, and pretty soon, I was running every day. I was feeling great and pounds started peeling off. Then I decided I wanted to be in control of what I put in my body."

The by-product of her running program was that she started looking at food differently, not as an emotional crutch. And she didn't want to put junk in her active body, which had begun crying out for high-caliber food. "It's just food. It's not my comforter. It's not going to make life's hassles go away. But it is fuel for my body."

Now Laura eats a healthful diet, made up of such foods as whole grains and fruit, tuna sandwiches, salads, chicken breasts, and vegetables. Laura lost 40 pounds, which she has kept off successfully for almost six years. Along the way, the memory of her mother's strength and courage battling the disease taught her the importance of appreciating the little things in life, every single day.

Laura is one of those people who bucked the trend of what every dieter already knows: It can be fairly easy to lose weight, but maintaining that loss is another, entirely

TRUTH

Meal planning keeps you on track.

Plan your meals, even if it's for only three days at a time. Meal planning gives you structure, helps guard against unplanned eating, and helps you stick to a healthy eating plan—and it keeps me from buying lots of snacks and unnecessary foods. We do try to keep shopping fun, though: We each get to pick one treat every time we go to the grocery store.

different challenge. Anyone who is overweight has probably dieted away and regained more than his or her whole body weight over the years. Laura is a testament to the fact that the cycle can be broken—for her and for all of us.

ANATOMY OF A MYTH

A discouraging statistic among the overweight and those who treat them is that 95 percent of people who lose weight regain it—and sometimes more of it—within a few months or years. You've heard that, too, right?

This 95 percent figure has been so widely quoted over the last four decades—in magazines, diet books, research papers, even at congressional hearings—that it has become diet doctrine. And it is the reason so many people approach dieting feeling totally hopeless.

This number was first suggested in a 1959 clinical study of only one hundred patients treated for obesity at a nutrition clinic at New York Hospital in the 1950s. Its authors, Dr. Albert Stunkard and Mavis McLaren-Hume, published a paper in which they concluded, "Most obese persons will not stay in treatment, most will not lose weight, and of those who do lose weight, most will regain it." In all fairness, the study was done at a time when everybody thought obesity was easy to treat. Their study showed that it was not.

The 95 percent figure was repeated so often that it came to be regarded as fact, when it is really only clinical lore. Obesity researchers say that no one has a handle on how many people lose weight, regain it, or keep it off. The true failure rate could be much better—or much worse. The fact is that we just don't know.

But here's something we do know: Contrary to popular myth, you can lose weight and keep it off. It's been the mission of the National Weight Control Registry to prove just that. The more than five thousand registry participants have maintained their weight loss of 30 pounds or more for at least six years. Many have done even better than that, maintaining, on average, a 67-pound weight loss for five years. Between 12 percent and 14 percent have maintained a loss of more than 100 pounds.

Is there some deep, dark secret that enabled these dieters to lose weight and keep it off? The answer lies not in complicated hocus-pocus but in a few easily understood principles that I know you have heard me say before: They ate less. They enjoyed healthier food. They exercised regularly.

But let's talk about you. You've spent months counting calories, munching on veggies and fruit, and taking long walks. Finally, you've achieved a healthy weight. Now, how can you avoid regaining the pounds you've worked so hard to shed?

TRUTH

Flatulence is a sign of a healthy diet.

Sure, gastric distress can be a sign of disease. When I have patients who complain of gas, I sympathize but add that this may be proof that they're eating a healthy diet. Someone rarely inconvenienced by gas may not be consuming enough fiber. Each of us generates a pint to two quarts of gas per day. The more vegetables you eat, the more gas you produce. The gassiest foods are legumes (beans, lentils, peas, and peanuts, for example), bran, and dried fruit, but all plant matter contributes. Meat, eggs, fat, alcohol, and refined sugars are innocent. Dairy products cause gas in those who have lactose intolerance, the inability to digest lactose, the sugar in milk. There's no harm in cutting out a few offending foods, but blanket avoidance of fruits and vegetables is a bad idea. Antigas medications may give relief. They don't require a prescription.

FOLLOW A LIVABLE DIET

Keep in mind that popular diets work for one simple reason: They limit the number of calories you eat. Remember, whether the calories come from cheesecake or carrot sticks, if they total fewer than 1,500 a day, you will lose weight. But you've got to make friends with that diet in order to stick to it. There really isn't any diet, whether it's a brand name or not, that's going to work for you over the long term unless you can live with it. You should follow a diet that you like and that you can stay with. But to keep the weight off—and stay healthy—you will need to boost your fruit, veggie, and complex-carbohydrate intake and consume no more than 20 to 30 percent of calories from fat.

Of course, even with such straightforward guidelines, portion control is still critical. Watch portion sizes, even when you're not trying to keep your weight off, and make sure you don't consume more than your body can burn. The old edict that one portion of meat should be the size of a tape cassette or a serving of rice should be no bigger than a fist still makes sense. To watch your portions without being punitive, prepare less food. Measure out foods instead of dumping in the whole box. Grill one chicken breast per person. Or try something I do in a pinch: if you're eating a frozen "diet" entrée with dimensions reminiscent of airline food, bolster it with salad and extra veggies so you won't be ravenous an hour later.

As long as you're working within some basic parameters—opting for monounsaturated and polyunsaturated fats over saturated and trans fats, focusing on lean proteins, picking whole grains over processed carbs, getting plenty of fruits and veggies, controlling your

TRUTH

Regular salad dressing helps your body absorb nutrients.

Fat-free salad dressing isn't always your best bet. Salad veggies are packed with terrific nutrients like lycopene and beta-carotene. But your body can't absorb these without a little help from fat. This doesn't mean you should drown your greens in gobs of salad dressing: A small amount of olive oil will be sufficient. Or you can add low-fat cheese, nuts, seeds, or avocado.

portions to some degree—you're on the right track. The idea is to make changes that you can live with for the rest of your life. View it as a whole new way of doing things, not a temporary arrangement.

BE A LITTLE FREER

Maintenance is like dieting, except that you can be a little freer. To determine just how liberal you can be, after you reach your weight-loss goal, add 100 calories to your diet every few days until your weight stabilizes.

Dieters in the registry still followed a low-fat, low-cal eating plan to maintain their weight loss, nearly 1,400 calories a day, with around 27 percent of their calories coming from fat. Very few of them eat a low-carb diet, and they eat four to five times a day. Some continue to use meal-replacement products for portion and calorie control to help them keep weight off. I wouldn't recommend having them too often, but in a pinch go for it.

TRUTH

Cutting 100 calories a day prevents weight gain.

Keeping pounds at bay requires a very small sacrifice, as little as 100 fewer calories a day—from eating less, exercising more, or a little of both. Small changes in behavior, such as fifteen extra minutes of walking per day or eating fewer bites at each meal, may be enough to stop weight gain, particularly those pounds we tend to gain in maintenance.

BE A FAITHFUL MEMBER OF THE BREAKFAST CLUB

If you're a breakfast skipper, vow to change. Over and over again, studies show that people who eat breakfast actually eat less on average than those who skip meals. Other evidence says breakfast eaters consume more vitamins and minerals and less cholesterol and fat, feel more energetic, have greater concentration, and can keep their weight in check. Plus, people who eat breakfast resist high-calorie foods better during the day, whereas those who don't eat breakfast make up for those "skipped calories" later owing to excessive hunger. Eating breakfast also boosts your physical and mental energy and helps keep it lifted throughout the day.

TRUTH

Being brown in color does not mean a bread is high in fiber.

While shopping in the bread aisle, don't assume that a brown loaf of bread is higher in natural fiber. That dark color is often courtesy of additives such as molasses, caramel coloring, or food dyes. If the bread's ingredient list states it contains whole wheat or other whole grains, it probably has fiber, but check the label for the number of grams of fiber per serving. Also, according to labeling regulations, manufacturers can use the term *whole wheat* when only 40 percent of the bread contains whole grain. Look for bread labeled "100 percent whole wheat," and you won't go wrong. Likewise, a loaf with seeds or oatmeal flakes gracing its top isn't necessarily high in fiber, either. Basically, they're just decoration.

So no matter how rushed you are in the morning, make it a point to eat breakfast, even if it's something you can grab quickly like a cup of yogurt and a piece of fruit. I confess that I've had to make peace with this health advice because I'm rarely ready for breakfast when I get up, but then I'm famished by 10 A.M. if I haven't eaten anything. I've learned that if I want to stay energized through the morning and beyond, I've got to eat at least a light breakfast.

ALLOW YOURSELF SOME TREATS

It is silly to deny yourself or feel guilty about food. I'm now a big believer in treating yourself—which is the basis of my Treat Yourself Diet that begins on page 237. Put more foods on your "okay to eat" list. Make a list of foods you covet most, and let yourself sample some regularly—a spoonful of ice cream, a handful of cashews. Scared you'll head straight for the ice cream and chow down until you've hit the bottom of the pint? Odds are firmly against it. When you let yourself eat certain foods, the urgency to have them in large quantities eventually dissipates. What has helped me keep my weight off is allowing myself some leeway. As long as I eat healthfully during the week, I can splurge a bit on weekends. Yes, I yearn for sweets—and my remedy is to freeze Halloween candy, namely, those tiny candy bars. Frozen, they take longer to eat, so I can savor every bite, and they're smaller, so I'm satisfied with less. And since they're packed away in the freezer, they're out of my sight.

TRUTH

Your taste buds get bored after the third bite.

Savor the first three bites of your food. By the fourth, your taste buds are bored. You don't need fifty bites of something delicious. Nor do you need the calories. If you can just enjoy those three bites, you won't bolt down the whole serving.

BE REALISTIC ABOUT THE SIZE YOU'LL KEEP IN MAINTENANCE

Often in our desire to lose weight we set unrealistic goals for ourselves. You may be able to attain airbrushed-girl fantasy weight, but what are the odds you'll stay there? The weight may come off, but we don't keep it off, since we cannot live with such a drastic dietary plan. Don't set yourself up for failure. Set a weight-loss goal of no more than 10 percent of your current body weight. That's what a panel of experts from the National Academy of Sciences recommends. (For example, a 150-pound woman should shoot for losing no more than 15 pounds.) If you can keep that much weight off for six months, then go for another 10 percent. If you aim too low, you may become frustrated with the deprivation involved, setting the stage for backsliding. If you try for a comfortable weight, though it may be somewhat heavier than you'd hoped, you'll be more likely to maintain it.

To my women readers: Don't base your goals around dress size. Unlike weight, which is a quantifiable figure you can measure, dress sizes have become frustratingly unpredictable. Not only is a size 6 today probably roomier than a size 6 from just a few years ago, different clothing brands have varying sizes of a size 6. Over the past several decades, the clothing industry latched onto a bankable truth: Women tend to feel better and buy more when we fit into a smaller size. Dress designers manipulate dress sizes—a tactic called vanity sizing—by actually adding extra inches of fabric to clothing without changing the number on the tag. For example, if you measure a size 10 pair of pants today, they might be as wide around the waist and hips as a size 16 from ten years ago. What this teaches us is to shoot for a comfortable weight, not a deceptively tiny dress size.

I've had to change my own outlook on size. I will never look like a model—it's not in my genes. Besides, I love going out for dinner and cooking. I'm not willing to give up these things to be thinner. Instead of dwelling on

TRUTH

Eating slowly fills you up and helps you eat less.

Eat slowly, and you'll help control your weight. Gobbling your food doesn't give your stomach the twenty minutes it needs to signal your brain that it's full, making it easy to unknowingly cram in more calories than you need. Instead of wolfing down a meal mindlessly, chew each mouthful mindfully, put down your utensils between bites, and pay attention to the flavors and textures. When you don't eat on autopilot, you naturally eat a little less, and you could cut out as many as 100 calories a day. That's all it takes to drop 10 pounds in a year. So give yourself at least twenty minutes to enjoy a meal.

the things that are "wrong" with your body, concentrate on the things that are right. Work with what you've got. Embrace what is healthy for you and attempt to maximize your own unique body type—and you've given yourself a great gift.

LOVE YOUR SCALE

We drag it out, dust it off, and step on it. That darn bathroom scale, it's got to be broken. We pick the thing up, shake it a couple of times, strip off rings, hair clips, anything, and step on it again. "Hmmm, that still can't be right," we mutter as the needle zooms.

The bathroom scale—we dread it, but it's really a dieter's best friend. Studies show that weighing yourself on a regular basis helps keep the pounds off. But you may want to refrain from doing it every day. The average weight loss for most diets is around 2 pounds a week, so you won't notice a difference weighing yourself day to day. And if you've been eating well all week and exercising, it can be disheartening to find you haven't lost any weight and make you more likely to ditch your diet. Our body weight fluctuates by up to 4 pounds in a day, mainly owing to what we eat, whether or not we have our period, and how hydrated we are.

Successful maintainers weigh themselves weekly, never allowing a gain of more than 5 pounds. To be successful at preventing a relapse, immediately take action when your weight increases, by modifying your diet or resuming your original one, stepping up your physical activity, or giving up treats or snacks until your weight goes down again. It's part of an ongoing vigilance that lets you keep conscious control over your weight. People who stop weighing themselves tend to put the pounds right back on.

Allow for small regains. Although a weight gain of 2 to 3 pounds can be blamed on water retention, a gain of 5 pounds or more means you need to take stock. (If you don't weigh yourself, use the fit of your clothes to gauge your progress.) Keeping your weight within a 5-pound range means you'll maintain a loss for good. I weigh myself every morning—but that's not for everyone.

I recommend weighing yourself once a week, in the morning, with an empty bladder and naked. This will give you the most accurate reading and will keep you on the right track. Besides using the scale, you could also take your waist and hip measurements to check your progress. Personally, I go by how my clothes fit. If I'm still on speaking terms with my jeans, then my weight is right where it should be.

KEEP TRACK OF WHAT YOU EAT

If you start gaining weight again, and you haven't recorded what you're eating, it's difficult to pinpoint what you're doing wrong. Periodically at least, try to keep tabs on your eating. Should your weight begin to creep up, write down everything you're eating to see where the extra calories are coming from. Because eating is often connected with stress, boredom, and the blues—even

TRUTH

Bland isn't always best for the digestive tract.

Myth has it that anyone with a sensitive stomach should stick to white foods such as rice, white bread, potatoes, and milk. The truth is that even spicy foods won't aggravate most digestive disorders, including ulcers, colitis, and irritable-bowel syndrome. Every digestive tract has quirks, so you are probably aware of which foods cause you trouble. Avoid whatever bothers you, but don't assume that bland meals are therapeutic.

happiness—documenting what you eat, and when, can also help you break bad habits. For instance, if you always reach for a box of cookies after a rough day at work, find other ways to decompress, such as calling a friend or taking a walk.

SEEK SUPPORT

It's tough to keep your weight down when everyone around you is eating ice cream. Patty, another good friend, has shed 75 pounds while raising two teenage sons. When she was recently struggling with an extra 10 pounds, she held a family meeting. "Please let's not have any more ice cream in the house; if you want some, I'll give you money to go out for it," she said. Her family agreed. Her husband and sons have also supported her by accepting the low-calorie meals she cooks for the family.

Plenty of studies underline the importance of support. One study, which appeared in the *Journal of the American Medical Association,* took a group of 1,032 overweight or obese adults who had lost weight using a diet focusing on fruits, vegetables, low-fat dairy products, and whole grains. Their average weight loss was 19 pounds. One group was given regular phone and in-person support from a counselor, another had unlimited access to a website designed to encourage weight-loss maintenance, and a third (the control group) received no support. After thirty months, all three groups had regained some weight, and the differences among the groups were small. But the personal contact group fared best, with a net loss of 9.2 pounds. The website users followed, with 7.3 pounds, and the control group brought up the rear (so to speak).

If you lose weight with the help of a group or a professional, continue to attend meetings. Staying in touch

TRUTH

"Perimeter shopping" is healthy shopping.

By "perimeter shopping," I'm talking about the outside borders of the grocery store. That's where you find the freshest fruits and vegetables, meats, fish, poultry, and low-fat dairy foods. It is in the inner aisles of the store where you'll encounter most processed, canned, and frozen foods. So stick mostly to the outside aisles, and you'll find foods with higher nutritional value.

with others in the same situation will strengthen your resolve.

PUT YOURSELF FIRST MORE OFTEN

I'm a working mom like everyone else—and I mean moms who work inside and outside of the home. I have a husband and three children. I love my life, but I do admit to taking less-than-perfect care of myself some of the time. So every now and then, I stop and say to myself, "Hey, if you want to live to be ninety and enjoy being ninety when you get there, you'd better slow down." Then I sit down and breathe, literally. I take ten slow deep breaths and plan how to squeeze a little more time for myself and my family out of the next few days. It's always a struggle to figure out how to get enough work done during the day, preserve the family sit-down dinner, and keep enough energy to devote to my husband's and children's needs. These are the balls in life that might not bounce back if I drop them once too often, and that is always in the back of my mind. But also in the back of my mind is the ball signifying my physical health and peace of mind. I know that if I drop that once too often, I might not come bouncing back, either.

If you're busy taking care of the family and have little time to yourself, it's tempting to put your health and fitness goals on the back burner. You've heard it before, but it bears repeating: To give to others, we have to learn to take care of ourselves. If we could show ourselves only a fraction of the affection and attention we give our families, we'd be so much better off. Find ways to make room for your needs. People I know who have lost weight and kept it off have developed a healthy sense of self-centeredness: They commit to setting aside time to do things they enjoy—getting a massage or going horseback riding, for example.

TAME EMOTIONAL OVEREATING FOR GOOD

Every once in a while I can feel a wave of the blues upon me. I can rarely pinpoint a cause—in fact, I no longer search for one. What used to throw me—and cause me to eat emotionally—I now welcome as a normal fluctuation of my psyche. I feel comfortable welcoming it because I don't expect it to stay. Over the years I've come to recognize these short-lived periods and use them to slow down and indulge myself—in short, to be a little selfish, spend time on myself, and spoil myself when I otherwise might not. It takes time to allow the indulgence, and it's not always easy with work and the kids, but I now consider these episodes way stations, and I think they make me healthier in the long run.

Make a point of noticing emotional triggers that make you want to eat—try writing them down. When they occur, grab a cool drink of water to give you a chance to think, and then begin an activity you've decided to substitute for eating, such as a fifteen-minute walk, calling a friend, reading a chapter of a book you enjoy, or using the computer.

TRUTH

Men keep emotions out of weight control.

There's a lot women can learn from men when it comes to losing weight and keeping it off. True, it's easier for guys. That's because men tend to be fat in their chests and bellies. And upper-body fat comes off far easier than lower-body fat. But there's more to the story.

First, men have less of a sweet tooth—they prefer meat—whereas women crave sugary snacks as comfort food. The protein in lean meat will fill you up, while sweet treats cause energy levels to spike and fall, leaving you hungry.

Second, men generally don't give in to stress eating. Do you automatically raid the fridge after a bad day at the office? A British study found that women are more likely than their male co-workers to seek out foods high in sugar and fat during stressful times.

Finally, men don't beat themselves up for blowing their diets. After a slip, women are likely to assuage their guilt with another binge, whereas men get right back on track. So close the gender gap, stay away from the sweets, and you can stay trim, too.

Self-Care Mantras

I'll just go for a walk.

I'll remember to breathe.

I'll go for a ride instead of watching TV.

I'll go to the movies instead of the ice-cream store.

I'll take a bath and let my spouse feed the kids.

I'll drink a glass of pure water on my coffee break.

I'll skip the second glass of wine.

I'll serve fruit for dessert.

I'll ask my spouse to take the kids to the park so I can get a massage.

I'll spend a little time dreaming.

I'll tell myself often that I am the love of my life.

TRUTH

There's a difference between biological hunger and emotional hunger.

For successful weight management, it's important to figure out if you're really hungry. A mild gnawing in the stomach, light-headedness, difficulty concentrating, and feeling faint are all signs of biological hunger. But you need to distinguish this from emotional hunger—that urge to eat mindlessly during times of stress. If hunger strikes between meals, drink a glass of water and wait ten minutes to see if it passes. Meanwhile, ask yourself if it's something other than food you need: a break from work, a breath of fresh air, or a nap.

REMIND YOURSELF OF WHY YOU LOST THE WEIGHT

One of the most difficult parts of maintenance is staying motivated, but one of the best ways to stay motivated is to remind yourself of what your life was like when you

TRUTH

Losing a few pounds can make a big difference to your health.

Some people think they'll never lose enough weight to improve their health. Not true! For example, for every 2 pounds of excess weight you lose, your blood cholesterol drops by an average of 3 points. That's nothing to scoff at. Losing weight can help your blood pressure, too. In one study, after losing as few as 9 pounds, people were able to bring their high blood pressure down to normal. Some people even went off medication, with their doctors' approval.

233

were heavy. Write this reminder down in a journal, or keep a few old photos of yourself around from when you were overweight. Take a look at both often; it will have a magical effect on your motivation.

KEEP YOUR REAR IN GEAR

You've heard it all before, I know, and it does get monotonous. You've been practically brainwashed regarding the health benefits of a consistent exercise program. It goes without saying that exercise will never be as easy as a chocolate éclair and a good book (or whatever your favorite pastime may be), but nonetheless we are going to have to get active, especially if we want to keep those pounds lost.

Exercise got you to your goal, and it will help you stay here. Data on maintainers show that they work out more than most other people—between sixty and ninety minutes a day. Walking is their number one exercise. Many wear pedometers and take 11,000 to 12,000 steps a day. That's equivalent to 5½ to 6 miles. Others combine walking with something that's more planned, like aerobic class, resistance training, biking, or swimming. All in all, women expend 2,545 calories a week; men expend 3,293 calories a week. And they watch only about ten hours of television a week—a third of what the typical American watches.

If you still consider exercise a chore, change the way you view working out. Close your eyes and think "Physical activity" but associate the thought with something physical you really enjoy doing. If you like shopping, the next time you're at the mall, walk around the complex a couple of times before you make your purchases. If you enjoy dancing, when you go to the club spend more time on the dance floor than you do sitting at a table. And, yes, getting physical with your significant other is exercise, too!

You just need to *increase movement* and be more physically active. When it comes to moving your body, think about all the benefits you receive from breaking a sweat: You'll lose weight and keep it off. You will improve your shape. You'll strengthen your bones, which can drastically reduce your risk for osteoporosis. You'll have more energy and less stress. When you work out, you are calmer and better able to cope with life. You'll lessen your risk of many illnesses. You'll be more productive and more likely to perform better on your job. You'll feel better about yourself and your self-confidence will increase. And exercise improves your sex life. With all of that, in this one instance, isn't it worth trying to hold on to what you lost?

EXTRA, EXTRA

Preferences for salty food are learned.

If you slowly cut down sodium intake, your desire for salt will decrease. Salt or sodium—call it whatever you want to. It can play a role in high blood pressure and is something you should keep an eye on. That's important because people with high blood pressure are more likely to develop heart disease and stroke. These diseases are the number one and number three killers in the United States today.

Old habits die hard, especially ones that have been around for eight thousand years. That's how long people have been adding salt to their food. While the easiest way to cut the salt is to toss out your shaker, that only accounts for 15 percent of the salt we consume. If you want or need to cut down on your sodium intake, here are some other ways to shake the habit:

- Cut back on high-sodium processed foods such as luncheon meats, processed cheese, hot dogs, chips, and canned products. Americans consume up to 75 percent of their sodium from processed foods.
- Experiment with the flavors of fresh herbs and spices and lemon juice. They can add a whole different taste to foods.
- Avoid seasoned salts such as onion, garlic, and celery salts.
- Read labels. Know what you're buying. Sodium may be hidden in chemical names such as sodium alginate, sodium sulfite, disodium phosphate, sodium benzoate, monosodium glutamate, and sodium citrate.
- At restaurants ask to have food prepared without salt. If you're careful about choosing and preparing food with little or no added salt, you can bring your intake way down.

Dr. Nancy Snyderman's Treat Yourself Diet

I have some wonderful news for you: You can drop 8 to 10 pounds this month without having to forfeit all the foods and drinks you love. I do not believe in denial and deprivation. I believe in moderation and surrounding yourself with nutritious foods. I also believe that deprivation is a great way to set yourself up for failure. And, finally, I believe in a little bit of planning. Good foods, the occasional treat, and some forethought can be the basis for a commonsense weight-loss plan. Personally, I allow myself a range of 2 to 3 pounds. But as soon as I see an extra 5 pounds on the scale I know it's time to swing into action. That's when I take the extra pounds seriously. Completely depriving yourself of your favorite foods guarantees you won't be on a losing streak for long. Deprivation works only temporarily until we've had enough, throw in the towel, and splurge until we can't eat any more. The solution? Try a new approach: Don't go hungry and enjoy a treat meal once a week.

All you have to do is follow my nutritious meal plan six days a week, and then take Saturday or Sunday to enjoy your favorite foods in moderation with a "treat meal." That way, you get to enjoy the foods you love, while still losing pounds and inches. Enjoying your favorite foods is the one ingredient that's missing from practically every single diet ever devised, yet it's the one ingredient that makes weight loss successful over the short and long terms. If you eliminate favorite foods from your diet, you will only want them more, which increases the chances that you won't stick to your plan.

This plan will provide healthy, tasty foods that make you feel satiated, so you'll never be hungry or tempted to overeat. There are no forbidden foods, which means you won't be constantly thinking about what you can't have.

At the same time, you'll be retraining yourself to enjoy wholesome foods. Accordingly, this plan is nutrient dense (rich in complex carbohydrates, lean meat, poultry, fish, low-fat dairy products, and fresh fruits and vegetables). Complex carbohydrates (legumes, whole grains, fruits, and vegetables) take longer to break down, providing lasting energy. They also add a dose of fiber, which absorbs water on its way through the digestive tract, making you feel fuller. Plus, it takes longer to chew most fibrous foods, slowing down the process of eating and giving your brain a chance to recognize the signs of satiety. Add protein to your meal, and the satisfaction you get will help you reach your goal.

HOW IT WORKS

On dieting days, you'll eat three delicious meals a day and two snacks. What will you eat? Proteins like meat, fish, chicken, eggs, and dairy foods like cheese. All sorts of vegetables and fruits. Even carbs like pasta and bread. Oils and salad dressings. A little wine on occasion, if you wish. And some fast food? Absolutely.

You'll personalize the diet by mixing and matching your meals and snacks from the lists that follow. You'll create each day's menu from lists of thirty breakfasts, thirty lunches, thirty dinners, and thirty snacks, according to what you enjoy eating. Each breakfast meal is calorically equivalent to every other on the same list. This is true for lunch, dinner, and snacks. You may select a different meal every day or repeat your favorites and stay at the same level. Base your selections on what you like to eat and your lifestyle. Not a fan of tuna? Skip it. Love oatmeal? Then have it every morning.

Unlike many diets, mine allows you enough latitude to adapt the plan to your tastes. I won't shoehorn you and everyone else into a "one size fits all" diet; instead, you'll have a wide range of meals, all of which can be prepared with products easily available in any supermarket.

The diet provides between 1,200 and 1,500 calories a day. That's enough to help you lose up to 10 pounds a month but not so low in calories that you're starving.

The Treat Yourself Diet simplifies your life, too. You won't have to do any laborious, obsessive counting of carbs, fat, calories, or fiber; nor is there any menu planning required or boring food lists. Everything is done for you. You'll find, too, that you're consistently satisfied by the food you're eating.

As I've said, no foods or food groups are restricted; only the portion sizes of the food you eat are regulated in order to stimulate your body to burn fat. Of course, before starting, talk to your doctor about how much weight you have to lose.

EASY-TO-FOLLOW GUIDELINES

Here are some ground rules to help you get the most from this plan.

- Drink mostly water when you're thirsty, but enjoy calorie-free beverages in moderation.
- Add flavor to food using herbs, spices, lemon or lime juice, bouillon, mustard, vinegar (any type), black pepper, light soy sauce, sugar substitutes, and Worcestershire sauce.
- Use measuring spoons, cups, or a food scale until you learn to eyeball portion sizes accurately. If you hate the idea of that, simply use your hand as a measuring device. Servings of protein are about the size of the palm of your hand; servings of vegetables, about the size of your fist; servings of good carbs like rice or whole wheat pasta, about the size of your cupped hand. For servings of fats, oils, and salad dressings, the size of your thumb equals a serving.
- At any meal, you can eat more vegetables (except starchy ones like potatoes and corn). For example,

add a cup of steamed green beans (22 calories) to dinner or a half cup of chopped romaine lettuce (4 calories) to a sandwich.

- Widen the color spectrum of fruits and vegetables you eat. Doing so is one of the simplest ways to ensure you follow a health-protective diet. Think deep colors and textures, and you immediately know which foods to choose. Blueberries, grape tomatoes, spinach, and even dark chocolate contain cancer-fighting antioxidants that destroy those nasty free radicals that are released during digestion. Sweet potatoes are considered to be at the top of the list, as they are loaded with vitamin C, fiber, and potassium. Apples, beans, kiwis, oranges, and any kind of grain such as brown rice or oats, all provide us with the vitamins and minerals that we need every day and can lower our cholesterol levels and strengthen our hearts. They are pure and simple foods that fight cancer and heart disease and also are proven to reduce the effects of aging.

- Use good fats and oils and butter or margarine, in moderation (up to 2 tablespoons a day). If you choose margarine, make sure it is free of trans fats. Choose monounsaturated fats (e.g., olive and canola oils, nuts and seeds) over those high in saturated or trans fats (e.g., fatty cuts of meat, full-fat dairy products, butter, french fries, cookies, crackers).

- Try specially manufactured foods, such as low-fat and low-sodium cheeses, low-fat frozen yogurt, and reduced-calorie salad dressings. If you like the taste, they can help you stick to your diet. But check their calorie counts, because these products can be a lot more calorically costly than you think if you're not careful.

- Use a nonstick pan so you can cook with minimal fat.
- Put your knowledge to practice. For instance, read product labels to help you select low-fat foods. And choose recipes that are lower in fat, sugar, and sodium than those you've been preparing.
- Because these meals aren't full of special "diet" foods, it's easy to share them with your family. If they aren't restricting their calories, just increase the portion sizes.
- Don't skip meals.
- Be careful at restaurants. Feel free to eat out, but remember that restaurant portions tend to be at least two to three times the standard serving size. Share appetizers and desserts and, if possible, an entrée. Stay away from supersized portions, such as giant 5-ounce bagels and heaping platters of pasta. If you're not sharing, don't feel compelled to clean your plate. Choose steamed, grilled, baked, or broiled items, and steer clear of sautéed and fried foods, dishes laden with cheese or cream sauces, and all-you-can-eat buffets. Eat slowly, enjoy the food, and don't waste calories on courses you don't absolutely love.
- Stay active. Regular activity is one of the most important factors in losing pounds and maintaining

a healthy weight. It's not lack of time that prevents exercise; it's really not. It's a matter of priorities. Move exercise to the top of your to-do list. Many people find they're more efficient when they exercise regularly. Exercise on as many days of the week as you can (five is ideal); aim for at least thirty minutes per session.

- Visualize your success several times a day. See your new, healthier body in your mind's eye. Envision yourself lean and lithe. Pull out some old photos of yourself when you were slimmer and tape them to the fridge or your home computer.

- Remind yourself of the health benefits of improving your diet. Studies have shown that those who truly believe a diet lower in fat and processed foods will improve their health are more likely to make the shift successfully.

- Make the Treat Yourself Diet a part of your lifestyle. (What's the downside? Feeling better?) If you want to manage your weight long term, you'll have to make changes that are opposite "going on a diet"—like treating yourself. Treating yourself to good health and a good long life. That doesn't sound so bad, does it? Now let's get started!

TREAT YOURSELF MEALS

These complete, modular meals give you a very simple way to support your weight loss. You don't have to count anything. As long as you select one breakfast, one lunch, one dinner, and two snacks daily, you'll have everything you need for healthy eating and steady weight loss.

Treat Yourself Breakfasts

1. 1 slice whole wheat toast
   1 teaspoon trans fat–free margarine (optional)
   1 poached, soft-boiled, or hard-boiled egg
   ½ grapefruit

2. ½ whole-grain bagel
   1 tablespoon reduced-fat cream cheese
   2 ounces lox
   ½ cup (4 ounces) orange juice

3. 1 cup cereal, high fiber (e.g., Bran Buds or Fiber One)
   1 cup (8 ounces) skim, 1%, or soy milk
   1 cup fresh berries

4. Whole wheat English muffin
   1 tablespoon jam
   1 piece fresh fruit (e.g., 1 peach, ¼ cantaloupe, ½ grapefruit, or 1 orange)

5. 1 cup (8 ounces) yogurt, plain, fat-free
   1 sliced banana
   1 tablespoon jam (to mix with yogurt)

6. 1 slice toaster french toast
   1 cup fresh berries
   1 tablespoon maple syrup

7. 1 slice whole wheat toast
   1 tablespoon peanut butter
   1 piece fresh fruit (e.g., 1 peach, ¼ cantaloupe,
   ½ grapefruit, or 1 orange)

8. 1 whole wheat English muffin
   2 slices Canadian bacon, cooked
   1 piece fresh fruit (e.g., 1 peach, ¼ cantaloupe,
   ½ grapefruit, or 1 orange)

9. Hot cereal, ¾ cup cooked
   1 cup skim, 1%, or soy milk
   1 cup berries

10. Smoothie on the run: vanilla nutritional beverage
    (e.g., Boost or Ensure) blended with 1 cup frozen
    fruit (unsweetened)

11. Cereal bar
    1 cup skim or 1% milk
    1 piece fresh fruit (e.g., 1 peach, ¼ cantaloupe,
    ½ grapefruit, or 1 orange)

12. 2 scrambled eggs, or 4 scrambled egg whites if you
    are watching your cholesterol
    2 slices turkey bacon, cooked
    1 cup fresh berries

13. Low-fat frozen pancakes, heated, 3 pieces
    1 tablespoon maple syrup
    1 cup sliced strawberries

14. 1 cup sugar-free fruit-flavored yogurt
    ½ cup low-sugar granola

1 piece fresh fruit (e.g., 1 peach, ¼ cantaloupe, ½ grapefruit, or 1 orange)

15. ½ cup low-fat or fat-free cottage cheese
1 cup pineapple chunks, fresh or canned in their own juice

16. 1 slice rye toast
1-ounce slice Swiss cheese
1 cup tomato juice

17. 2 scrambled egg whites
2 slices Canadian bacon, cooked
½ cup orange juice

18. 1 slice whole-grain toast
2 turkey sausage patties
½ grapefruit

19. 1 slice whole-grain toast
Omelet: 1 whole egg, 1 egg white, ½ cup chopped vegetables (onion, green pepper, mushrooms)—cooked in 1 teaspoon olive oil
1 fresh orange

20. ¾ cup cooked Cream of Wheat
1 cup skim, 1%, or soy milk
1 cup fresh berries

21. 1 medium (2½-inch diameter) bran muffin
½ cup (4 ounces) grapefruit or orange juice

22. ½ whole-grain bagel
1 hard-boiled egg

1 piece fresh fruit (e.g., 1 peach, ¼ cantaloupe, ½ grapefruit, or 1 orange)

23. Soy smoothie: 1 cup soy milk blended with 1 cup frozen fruit (unsweetened)
1 cereal bar

24. 1 cup yogurt mixed with ½ cup high-fiber cereal
1 cup blueberries

25. ¾ cup oat bran cooked with 1 cup skim milk, topped with 2 teaspoons raisins and a sprinkle of cinnamon
¼ cantaloupe

26. Smoothie: Blend together 1 cup berries (any type), 8 ounces light yogurt, and 4 ounces skim milk.
1 slice whole wheat bread spread with 2 teaspoons peanut butter

27. ½ cup low-fat calcium-fortified cottage cheese
1 slice whole wheat toast, with 1 teaspoon butter
¼ cantaloupe

28. 1 whole wheat waffle
1 tablespoon all-fruit jam
1 tangerine
1 cup skim, 1%, or soy milk

29. 1 medium apple, sliced
1 tablespoon peanut butter
2 slices turkey bacon, cooked

30. 2 large shredded wheat biscuits
    1 sliced banana
    1 cup skim, 1%, or soy milk

Treat Yourself Lunches

1. Chicken Caesar salad: 3 ounces grilled chicken
   breast, cut into pieces, over 2 cups romaine lettuce
   with 2 tablespoons light Caesar dressing and
   2 tablespoons croutons

2. 1 bowl vegetable soup (about 1½ cups)
   5 whole wheat crackers
   1 cup mixed chopped fruit

3. Tuna sandwich: 3 ounces tuna mixed with
   1 tablespoon mayonnaise on 2 slices whole wheat
   bread and 1 slice fresh tomato

4. Pita sandwich: 1 whole wheat pita filled with
   chopped lettuce and tomato, 1 ounce feta cheese,
   and 1 tablespoon Italian salad dressing
   10 baby carrots

5. 1 frozen low-fat pizza
   1 to 2 cups tossed mixed salad with 2 tablespoons
   reduced-fat dressing

6. 12 peel and eat shrimp (boiled)
   ¼ cup cocktail sauce
   ½ cup coleslaw (you can prepare a low-fat version
   by mixing a bag of coleslaw with reduced-fat
   coleslaw dressing)

7. Ham sandwich: 2 slices reduced-fat ham, 1-ounce
   slice Swiss cheese, and 1 teaspoon Dijon mustard
   on 2 slices whole-grain bread
   1 medium apple

8. Black bean burritos: ½ cup cooked black beans
   divided between and served in 2 low-carb tortillas,
   topped with a few tablespoons of chopped
   vegetables (green peppers, onions, tomatoes, etc.)
   and 2 tablespoons salsa

9. 4 ounces baked salmon
   1 cup steamed, boiled, or microwaved spinach
   ½ cup cooked brown rice

10. 4-ounce hamburger with sliced onion, tomato, and
    lettuce on 1 whole wheat hamburger bun
    1 to 2 cups tossed mixed salad with 2 tablespoons
    reduced-fat dressing

11. 1 bowl ready-to-eat chili
    1 to 2 cups tossed mixed salad with 2 tablespoons
    reduced-fat dressing

12. Peanut butter and jelly sandwich: 2 tablespoons
    peanut butter and 1 tablespoon jelly on 2 slices
    whole wheat bread
    1 medium apple

13. Greek salad: Toss together 2 ounces reduced-fat
    feta cheese, 2 cups romaine lettuce, and ½ cup
    each tomato, cucumber, and roasted red peppers.
    Top with 2 tablespoons light vinaigrette dressing.
    2 whole wheat crackers

14. Grilled cheese sandwich: Place 2 light cheese singles and 2 slices tomato on 2 slices whole wheat bread and cook in pan sprayed lightly with vegetable spray.
   1 cup baby carrots

15. Turkey sandwich: 2 ounces turkey breast, 1 teaspoon light mayonnaise, 2 to 3 tomato slices, lettuce or baby spinach leaves, and 1 teaspoon mustard on 2 slices light whole wheat bread
   1 cup light yogurt (any flavor)
   1 apple or piece of fresh fruit

16. Spinach salad: Toss baby spinach leaves with 1 sliced hard-boiled egg, 2 strips cooked turkey bacon, chopped raw mushrooms, and 2 tablespoons light salad dressing.
   1 medium pear or apple

17. Vegetarian sandwich: 1/4 mashed avocado, 1-ounce slice Swiss or Jarlsberg cheese, broccoli florets, and tomato slices on 2 slices light whole wheat bread
   1 cup fresh berries or 1 peach

18. Chef's salad: Top salad greens with 2 ounces extra-lean ham, turkey breast, or chicken breast, cut into strips; 1-ounce slice of Swiss cheese, cut into strips; tomato wedges; cucumber and onion slices; and 2 tablespoons reduced-fat salad dressing.
   1 medium apple or pear

19. 1 bowl prepared Manhattan clam chowder
    5 whole wheat crackers
    1 to 2 cups tossed mixed salad with 2 tablespoons
    reduced-fat dressing

20. Salade Niçoise: Place 3 ounces water-packed tuna,
    chilled green beans, 2 small chilled new potatoes,
    and 3 black olives on a bed of lettuce; drizzle with
    2 tablespoons light vinaigrette dressing.

21. Mexican veggie wrap: Layer 2 low-carb flour
    tortillas with 1 cup torn spinach leaves, 2 ounces
    Cheddar cheese, ½ cup canned black beans (rinsed
    and drained), ⅓ avocado, and 2 tablespoons salsa;
    eat cold or warmed slightly.

22. ½ cup hummus spread on cucumber slices
    1 medium apple

23. Roast beef sandwich: Spread 2 teaspoons Dijon
    mustard on 2 slices rye bread. Layer 4 ounces
    thinly sliced lean roast beef with tomato and onion
    slices between bread.

24. Stuffed potato: Top 1 large baked potato with
    ¼ cup grated cheese, 2 tablespoons low-fat sour
    cream, and 1 tablespoon chopped chives.

25. 1 frozen low-fat lasagna entrée,
    1 to 2 cups tossed mixed salad with 2 tablespoons
    reduced-fat dressing

26. Tomato stuffed with crab salad: Mix 4 ounces lump
    crabmeat with 1 tablespoon light mayonnaise and

2 tablespoons chopped celery. Serve on a generous
bed of lettuce.
1 medium apple

27. 1 low-fat turkey dog on hot dog roll with
mustard
½ cup baked beans
1 sliced tomato

28. 4 ounces grilled or baked chicken
1 cup steamed vegetables
1 to 2 cups tossed mixed salad with 2 tablespoons
reduced-fat dressing

29. Veggie burger: Place heated veggie burger on
whole wheat hamburger bun with a few tomato
slices, onion slices, lettuce, and mustard.
1 medium apple or pear

30. Grilled veggie salad: Place grilled or steamed
vegetables (zucchini, red bell peppers, onions,
string beans, etc.) on a bed of lettuce. Sprinkle
with reduced-fat feta cheese and drizzle with
2 tablespoons reduced-fat salad dressing.
1 cup chopped fresh fruit

Treat Yourself Dinners

1. Baked white fish: Top a 6-ounce white-flesh fish
(such as flounder, sole, or snapper) with 1
tablespoon Parmesan cheese and 2 teaspoons dried
bread crumbs. Sprinkle with paprika, salt, and
pepper; then spray with cooking spray. Bake in a

preheated 450°F oven until fish is opaque
throughout and flakes easily with a fork.
1 medium baked sweet potato
1 cup steamed vegetables such as asparagus, wax
beans, broccoli, or cauliflower

2. Low-fat pasta: In a nonstick skillet, cook 3 ounces
   ground turkey; add 1 cup cooked broccoli florets
   and ½ cup low-fat spaghetti sauce. Heat through.
   Toss with ½ cup cooked whole wheat spaghetti.
   Sprinkle with 1 tablespoon Parmesan cheese.
   1 to 2 cups tossed mixed salad with 2 tablespoons
   reduced-fat dressing

3. Grilled turkey burgers: In a bowl, combine 6
   ounces ground turkey, 2 tablespoons chopped
   onion, ½ teaspoon chopped garlic clove, and a
   dash of black pepper; mix well. Shape into 1 patty
   and grill or broil. Serve on whole wheat
   hamburger bun.
   ½ cup coleslaw (you can prepare a low-fat version
   by mixing a bag of coleslaw with reduced-fat
   coleslaw dressing)

4. 12 steamed shrimp
   1 medium baked potato topped with 1 tablespoon
   fat-free sour cream
   1 cup steamed spinach

5. 4 ounces roasted pork tenderloin
   ½ baked acorn squash
   1 to 2 cups tossed mixed salad with 2 tablespoons
   reduced-fat dressing

6. 4 ounces broiled or grilled flank steak
   1 medium baked sweet potato
   1 cup steamed zucchini

7. 4 ounces grilled or broiled salmon, prepared with
   1 teaspoon olive oil
   1 cup green beans, steamed
   1 medium baked potato topped with 1 tablespoon
   fat-free sour cream or 1 teaspoon butter

8. Beef and vegetable stir-fry: In 2 teaspoons hot
   sesame oil, cook 4 ounces thinly sliced lean beef
   until lightly browned. Add ½ cup cut-up broccoli;
   ¼ cup snow peas; and 2 tablespoons each bamboo
   shoots, sliced water chestnuts, and chopped onion.
   Cover and cook until beef loses its pink color and
   vegetables are tender-crisp, 7 to 10 minutes.
   ½ cup cooked brown rice

9. 4 ounces roasted turkey breast
   1 medium baked sweet potato
   1 cup green beans, steamed
   1 small whole-grain roll

10. Rice and beans: Combine ¾ cup drained canned
    black or pinto beans, ½ cup drained canned corn,
    ¾ cup canned stewed tomatoes, and a splash of
    hot pepper sauce (optional). Heat and serve over
    ½ cup cooked brown rice.

11. Spaghetti squash primavera: Prepare the squash
    by microwaving or baking. Sauté 1 cup cooked
    squash in 1 tablespoon olive oil with ½ cup

broccoli, ¼ cup chopped red pepper, and
2 tablespoons chopped onion. Top with heated
⅓ cup low-fat marinara sauce and 1 tablespoon
grated Parmesan cheese.

12. 2 medium broiled lamb chops
½ cup cooked brown rice
1 cup steamed yellow squash
1 to 2 cups tossed mixed salad with 2 tablespoons
reduced-fat dressing

13. 1 bowl vegetarian chili
5 whole wheat crackers
1 to 2 cups tossed mixed salad with 2 tablespoons
reduced-fat dressing

14. Scallops: Coat 8 ounces scallops with 2
tablespoons plain dried bread crumbs. In 1½
teaspoons olive oil, cook scallops, ⅓ cup chopped
onion, and 1 minced garlic clove for about 4
minutes, or until the scallops are opaque
throughout. Stir in 1 medium tomato, chopped.
Cover and cook for 1 minute. Serve over 2 cups
boiled and well-drained spinach.

15. Fast-food dinner: 1 cheeseburger or grilled chicken
sandwich
1 side salad with 2 tablespoons reduced-fat dressing
1 medium diet soda

16. 1 frozen low-fat entrée, steak tips Dijon
1 to 2 cups tossed mixed salad with 2 tablespoons
reduced-fat dressing

17. Kebab dinner: On 14-inch all-metal skewer, alternately thread 4 ounces beef or pork tenderloin cut into 5 chunks with 5 bite-size chunks zucchini and 5 cherry tomatoes. Baste with a mixture of 1 teaspoon balsamic vinegar, ½ teaspoon olive oil, and 1 minced garlic clove. Broil or grill, turning once, until meat is cooked through. Serve over ½ cup cooked brown rice or couscous.

18. 4 ounces baked chicken thighs, skinless
    1 cup steamed vegetables
    1 to 2 cups tossed mixed salad with 2 tablespoons reduced-fat dressing

19. 1 slice meat loaf (about 4 ounces)
    ½ cup mashed potatoes
    ½ cup cooked carrots
    1 cup steamed string beans

20. 4 ounces beef, eye of the round
    1 cup zucchini, sautéed with 1 teaspoon olive oil
    1 medium baked potato with 1 tablespoon fat-free sour cream

21. ½ cup pinto beans topped with salsa and chopped scallions, jalapeño peppers, or green bell peppers
    ½ cup brown rice
    Fresh tomato-basil salad: 1 sliced tomato, 2 ounces fresh part-skim mozzarella cheese, and 4 basil leaves, drizzled with 1 tablespoon vinaigrette dressing

22. 4 ounces filet mignon
    1 medium baked potato with 1 tablespoon fat-free sour cream
    1 tossed salad with 1 tablespoon salad dressing

23. 1 frozen reduced-fat entreé, pizza
    1 tossed salad with 1 tablespoon salad dressing

24. 1 baked Cornish hen
    ½ cup mashed sweet potatoes
    ½ cup cooked peas
    1 tossed salad with 1 tablespoon vinaigrette dressing

25. 4 ounces grilled tuna steak
    1 medium baked potato with fat-free sour cream
    1 cup steamed vegetables

26. 4 ounces roast chicken breast
    1 cup cooked carrots
    1 cup steamed brussels sprouts

27. Turkey cutlet: Lightly sprinkle both sides of a 4-ounce cutlet with salt and pepper. In a large nonstick skillet with lid, over medium-high heat, sauté turkey in ½ tablespoon olive oil for 5 to 7 minutes per side or until no longer pink in center.
    1 medium baked yam
    1 cup steamed broccoli or other green vegetable

28. Eggplant Parmesan: I don't usually make this recipe for just myself; it serves 4. You can serve your family, or if cooking for one, simply store the leftovers.

Preheat oven to 400°F. In a shallow dish, beat 2 egg whites and 2 tablespoons water until foamy. Dip eggplant slices into egg whites, then into bread crumbs, pressing the crumbs into the eggplant. Place eggplant on a baking sheet sprayed with vegetable spray. Then lightly spray vegetable cooking spray over eggplant slices. Bake 30 minutes, turning eggplant over after 20 minutes, until golden brown and cooked through. Cover with 1 cup low-fat spaghetti sauce; sprinkle ½ cup part-skim mozzarella and ¼ cup grated Parmesan cheese on top and bake for 20 minutes, or until eggplant is piping hot and sauce is bubbly. Serves 4.

1 tossed salad with 1 tablespoon salad dressing

29. Tacos: In a saucepan, brown 1 pound of ground turkey. Add one envelope of taco seasoning and cook according to package directions. (For vegetarian tacos, use 2 cans undrained black beans and one envelope of taco seasoning.) Serve with chopped tomatoes, chopped onions, salsa, and reduced-fat cheese as toppings (2 tablespoons per taco). Makes 3 servings (3 filled tacos per serving). Side dish: ½ cup cooked pinto beans

30. 4 ounces roast turkey breast
1 cup mashed butternut squash
1 cup steamed broccoli, green beans, or other green vegetable
1 small whole wheat dinner roll with 1 teaspoon butter

Treat Yourself Snacks

1. 1 ounce hard or semisoft cheese (Cheddar, Brie, Swiss, Gouda) with 5 whole wheat crackers
2. 1 piece of fresh fruit or 1 cup chopped fresh fruit
3. 1 cup fat-free, sugar-free yogurt
4. ½ cup fat-free ice cream or frozen yogurt
5. One 4-ounce fat-free pudding snack
6. 12 roasted almonds
7. 3 cups light popcorn
8. 3 graham cracker squares
9. 1 cup cappuccino made with skim milk
10. 1 cup instant hot cocoa prepared with skim milk or soy milk
11. 5 ounces white or red wine, 12 ounces beer, or 1 ounce hard liquor
12. 2 frozen fruit juice bars
13. 1 reduced-fat fudge bar, ice-cream sandwich, or ice-cream cone
14. 50 very thin pretzel sticks
15. 2 fig bars
16. ½ cup sorbet (100 to 130 calories per serving)
17. 3 California roll pieces with light soy sauce and wasabi
18. 10 baked corn chips with salsa
19. 12 mini barbecue-flavor rice cakes
20. 20 roasted peanuts
21. ¼ cup hummus with celery sticks
22. 5 reduced-fat whole wheat crackers with 1 ounce Jarlsberg or Cheddar cheese
23. 1 cup (8 ounces) carrot juice or vegetable juice

24. 1 half whole wheat English muffin spread with 2 teaspoons hazelnut chocolate spread
25. 2 ounces reduced-fat Cheddar cheese, 1 cup chopped raw vegetables
26. 3 graham cracker squares spread with 1 tablespoon peanut butter
27. 1 cup soy milk
28. Raw chopped veggies with 3 tablespoons reduced-fat dip
29. ½ cup reduced-fat cottage cheese with 1 peach, sliced
30. 1 square of dark chocolate

Your Treat Day

As crazy as it might sound, part of your success in following this plan is learning how to eat your favorite foods—stuff such as pie, cake, or pizza that doesn't usually fit the parameters of any program. I am a realist, and I know that no one can stick to a rigid diet program all the time without falling off the wagon. If I feel like I am being held hostage to one particular way of eating, I will quit. Here, you get the best of both worlds—by including a treat meal once a week. And guess what? You will still lose weight!

If you want to treat yourself to your favorite piece of cake once a week, more power to you—you aren't going to wreck your diet. Realistically, you can't have a slice of cake (which is about 500 calories or more) every night; instead, have a "treat meal." To keep you motivated, you're allowed some of your favorite foods in moderation. Looking forward to eating something you really enjoy, such as a slice of pie, is one of life's small pleasures. When you want a treat, have it and enjoy every bite. Then, forget it. Just don't have seconds! Oftentimes, when you fight your urge to eat something you really want, your strategy backfires. You may end up eating twice as much of another food, plus what you wanted all along.

Sample Food Plan

Here is an example of how you might plan seven days of eating, using these modular meal lists.

Monday

Breakfast
  1 slice whole wheat toast
  1 teaspoon trans fat–free margarine (optional)
  Poached, soft-boiled, or hard-boiled egg
  ½ grapefruit

Midmorning Snack
  1 cup fat-free, sugar-free yogurt

Lunch
  Chicken Caesar salad (page 248)

Midafternoon Snack
  1 piece of fresh fruit or 1 cup chopped fresh fruit

Dinner
  12 steamed shrimp
  1 medium baked potato topped with 1 tablespoon
    fat-free sour cream
  1 cup steamed spinach

Tuesday

Breakfast
   1 cup cereal, high fiber (e.g., Bran Buds)
   1 cup (8 ounces) skim, 1%, or soy milk
   1 cup fresh berries

Midmorning Snack
   ½ cup reduced-fat cottage cheese with 1 peach, sliced

Lunch
   Tuna sandwich (page 248) with 1 sliced fresh tomato

Midafternoon Snack
   ½ cup sorbet (or save for dessert with dinner)

Dinner
   1 low-fat frozen entrée, steak tips Dijon
   1 to 2 cups tossed mixed salad with 2 tablespoons
      reduced-fat dressing

Wednesday

Breakfast
   Smoothie on the run (page 245)

Midmorning Snack
   2 frozen fruit bars

Lunch
   Chef's salad (page 250)
   1 medium or large apple

Midafternoon Snack
   ¼ cup hummus with celery sticks

Dinner

　Rice and beans (page 254) over ½ cup cooked brown
　　rice

Thursday

Breakfast

　1 slice whole wheat toast
　1 poached, soft-boiled, or hard-boiled egg
　½ grapefruit

Midmorning Snack

　1 cup carrot juice or vegetable juice

Lunch

　1 bowl vegetable soup (about 1½ cups)
　5 whole wheat crackers
　1 cup mixed chopped fruit

Midafternoon Snack

　1 reduced-fat fudge bar, ice-cream sandwich, or
　　ice-cream cone (or save for dessert after dinner)

Dinner

　Baked white fish (page 252)
　1 medium baked sweet potato
　1 cup steamed vegetables, such as asparagus, wax
　　beans, broccoli, or cauliflower

Friday

Breakfast

　1 cup cereal, high fiber (e.g., Bran Buds)
　1 cup skim, 1%, or soy milk
　1 cup fresh berries

Midmorning Snack
  1 piece of fresh fruit or 1 cup chopped fresh fruit

Lunch
  Roast beef sandwich

Midafternoon Snack
  10 baked corn chips with salsa

Dinner
  4 ounces baked chicken thighs, skinless
  1 cup steamed vegetables
  1 to 2 cups tossed mixed salad with 2 tablespoons
    reduced-fat dressing

Saturday

Breakfast
  Smoothie on the run (page 245)

Midmorning Snack
  12 roasted almonds

Lunch
  Grilled cheese sandwich (page 250)

Midafternoon Snack
  5 whole wheat crackers with 1 ounce Jarlsberg or
    Cheddar cheese

Treat Dinner
  Sirloin steak (Since you're treating yourself, amounts
    do not matter. Be sensible, however. Six to eight
    ounces of steak is prudent.)
  1 medium baked potato with sour cream and butter

Salad with dressing
1 glass wine or 1 cocktail
1 slice of cheesecake

Sunday

Breakfast
. 1 cup cereal, high fiber (e.g., Bran Buds)
1 cup (8 ounces) skim, 1%, or soy milk
1 cup fresh berries

Midmorning Snack
3 graham cracker squares spread with 1 tablespoon
    peanut butter

Lunch
Greek salad (page 249)

Midafternoon Snack
2 frozen fruit juice bars (or save for dessert for
    dinner)

Dinner
Taco dinner (page 258)
½ cup pinto beans

CUSTOMIZING YOUR FOOD PLAN

If you'd like even more flexibility—and don't want to
stick to printed meal plans—you can customize the Treat
Yourself Diet even more. Do this by creating your own
breakfasts, lunches, dinners, and snacks, using my modular approach. Consult a calorie-counting book and come

up with breakfasts that total 250 to 300 calories; lunches and dinners, around 400 calories; and snacks, around 100 calories. You can add these to my selections for even more variety.

As you design your own "modules," keep them healthy. For example:

- Choose mostly whole grains like brown rice, whole wheat breads, and oatmeal, for example, overprocessed foods like white bread and baked goods. Have one of these "good" carbs with most meals.
- Don't ease up on vegetables! Enjoy generous servings of fresh or cooked low-calorie vegetables and salads.
- Stock up on fresh fruit. Fruit is not only filling but filled with nutrients and fibers. Make it your main choice for snacks and desserts.
- Choose healthy sources of proteins. That means proteins are lean, such as fish, poultry, and lean meats, as well as those containing heart-healthy unsaturated fats (like salmon, nuts, and soy).
- Go vegetarian once in a while. Have meatless meals on occasion, consisting of beans and other nutritious veggies.
- For convenience on busy days, replace home-cooked meals with low-fat frozen entrées. There are some delicious products out there and they make portion control a snap. These foods generally provide 350 calories a serving, so pair them

with a salad or fruit for dessert and you've got your 400-calorie meal.

ONE LAST THOUGHT

After giving birth to two children (one of my three is adopted), and being in my fifties, I don't have a perfect body, but I don't have a lot of complaints, either. Sure, sometimes it's a hassle finding clothes that fit me, but I wouldn't trade my curves for anything. These days, thankfully, rather than making a mental checklist of what is wrong with my body, I make one of what is right. Then I build on it. I replace any tendency I may have to complain with a resolve to encourage myself to do better and be better.

We must learn to love our bodies. Research suggests that men and women who are dissatisfied with their bodies are more likely to suffer anxiety and depression and engage in unhealthy habits such as overeating, binge eating, exercise avoidance, and alcohol consumption.

Fortunately, there is a lot you can do to start loving yourself more. It can begin with simple pampering. After I wrote this book, I took a few days to unwind and give myself some "me time." I'm a big believer in treating yourself with little luxuries . . . scented candles, sheets that feel good against your body, a refreshing facial, or just a nap because you feel like lounging. When I'm in pampering mode, I treat myself to regular pedicures and manicures. Find the pampering ideas that make you feel wonderful and just do them! These will help you reconnect with your body and begin the process of appreciating it more. They can be simple and don't have to be expensive; they just have to be all about you.

Try not to let your shape, or your appraisal of it, run your life. This is what I say to my children: "Would you let someone else criticize your looks the same way you do?" Spend more time complimenting yourself. It may be hard at first, and if you're stumped, ask a loving friend or your spouse to help you enumerate all your wonderful points. And don't be afraid to spend time looking at yourself naked in the mirror. Try describing ("my thighs are muscular") rather than judging ("my thighs are big and fat"). See yourself as a happy, healthy person who has achieved and mastered so much of what is important in this world. And when body parts "work," they are beautiful just because of that.

Your body is so much more than its outward appearance. I like to focus on how well my body functions—the energy I have, the ability it gives me to ride my beloved horses, the physical and emotional pleasure it gives to me to enjoy life. I learned to value my body when I became aware of the hard work it is doing for me every day, every hour, every second of my life. Whether I'm taking a walk, doing the dishes, hiking, or driving, I thank my body for carrying me, pulling me, lifting me, and giving me the ability to help and love others. My body doesn't betray me as long as I treat it in a loving way. So make a pact to stop body bashing and start appreciating your abilities, mind, talents, and wit—start acknowledging all that is strong and wonderful within you.

Once I started appreciating the hard work my body

does for me, I stopped treating it so poorly. I recognized that it needs and deserves good treatment for loyal service. Respecting your body boils down to five simple things. Sleep enough, eat healthily, don't smoke, exercise daily, relax, and have a partnership with a doctor during the good times.

Start every day with the reminder that, yes, you are beautiful or handsome, and you're wonderful. List all the miraculous things about your body on Post-it notes and stick one on your bathroom mirror, refrigerator, or dashboard each day.

So be good to your body—and your body will be good to you. If you learn to love yourself, the quest to be trim, fit, and healthy will be yours automatically, a gift you give yourself and something you very much deserve.

Resources

American Diabetes Association
ATTN: National Call Center
1701 North Beauregard St.
Alexandria, VA 22311
800-DIABETES or 800-342-2383
www.diabetes.org
The American Diabetes Association publishes many books and resources for health professionals and people with diabetes, including *Diabetes Forecast,* a monthly magazine for patients, and the journals *Diabetes, Diabetes Care,* and *Diabetes Spectrum.*

American Dietetic Association
120 South Riverside Plaza
Suite 2000
Chicago, IL 60606
800-877-1600
www.eatright.org

The American Dietetic Association is a professional organization that can help you locate a registered dietitian in your community.

American Heart Association

7272 Greenville Ave.

Dallas, TX 75231

800-aha-usa-1 or 800-242-8721

www.americanheart.org

The American Heart Association is a private voluntary organization that distributes literature on heart disease and its prevention. Local affiliates can be found on the organization's website.

American Society of Bariatric Physicians

2821 South Parker Rd., Suite 625

Aurora, CO 80014

303-770-2526

www.asbp.org

The mission of the American Society of Bariatric Physicians is to advance and support the physician's role in treating overweight patients. The society offers information on the growing problem of obesity, tips on weight loss, and a physician finder to help you locate a bariatric surgeon in your area.

Centers for Disease Control and Prevention

1600 Clifton Rd. NE

Atlanta, GA 30333

800-cdc-info or 800-232-4636

www.cdc.gov

The mission of the Centers for Disease Control and Prevention is to promote health and quality of life by preventing and controlling disease, injury, and disability. You'll find current information on diet and weight control on its website.

Federal Trade Commission, Diet & Fitness
www.ftc.gov/bcp/conline/edcams/fitness/coninfo.html
The website provides consumer information on topics such as finding the right weight-loss program and avoiding deception.

National Institutes of Health
9000 Rockville Pike
Bethesda, MD 20892
301-496-4000
www.nih.gov
The National Institutes of Health (NIH), a part of the U.S. Department of Health and Human Services, is the primary federal agency for conducting and supporting medical research. NIH scientists investigate ways to prevent disease as well as the causes, treatments, and even cures for common and rare diseases. Composed of 27 institutes and centers, the NIH provides leadership and financial support to researchers in every state and throughout the world.

National Institute of Mental Health
Science Writing, Press, and Dissemination Branch
6001 Executive Blvd., Room 8184, MSC 9663
Bethesda, MD 20892
301-443-4513 or 866-615-6464
www.nimh.nih.gov
The National Institute of Mental Health is the largest scientific organization in the world dedicated to research focused on the understanding, treatment, and prevention of mental disorders and the promotion of mental health.

National Stroke Foundation
9707 E. Easter Ln.
Centennial, CO 80112
800-STROKES or 800-787-6537
www.stroke.org

The National Stroke Foundation makes available to doctors and patients important information and tools for the prevention and treatment of stroke.

The National Weight Control Registry
Brown Medical School / The Miriam Hospital
Weight Control and Diabetes Research Center
196 Richmond St.
Providence, RI 02903
800-606-NWCR or 800-606-6927
www.nwcr.ws
The National Weight Control Registry (NWCR), established in 1994 by Rena Wing, Ph.D., from Brown Medical School, and James O. Hill, Ph.D., from the University of Colorado, is the largest investigation of long-term successful weight-loss maintenance. The NWCR was developed to identify and investigate the characteristics of individuals who have succeeded at long-term weight loss. The NWCR is tracking over five thousand individuals who have lost significant amounts of weight and kept it off for long periods of time. The National Weight Control Registry is not a weight-loss treatment program.

The Obesity Society
8630 Fenton St.
Suite 814
Silver Spring, MD 20910
301-563-6526
www.obesity.org
The Obesity Society is the leading scientific society dedicated to the study of obesity. Since 1982, the society has been committed to encouraging research on the causes and treatment of obesity, and to keeping the medical community and public informed of new advances.

Weight-Control Information Network
1 WIN Way
Bethesda, MD 20892
202-828-1025 or 877-946-4627
win.niddk.nih.gov/index.htm
The Weight-control Information Network provides the general public, health professionals, the media, and Congress with up-to-date, science-based information on weight control, obesity, physical activity, and related nutritional issues.

Selected References

Myth #1: Your Weight Is Your Fault

Christakis, N. A., and J. H. Fowler. 2007. The spread of obesity in a large social network over 32 years. *New England Journal of Medicine* 357:370–379.

Ebbeling, C. B., et al. 2007. Effects of a low-glycemic load vs. low-fat diet in obese young adults: A randomized trial. *Journal of the American Medical Association* 297:2092–2102.

Gundersen, C., et al. 2008. Food security, maternal stressors, and overweight among low-income US children: Results from the National Health and Nutrition Examination Survey (1999–2002). *Pediatrics* 122:e529–540.

Neumark-Sztainer, D., et al. 2008. Family meals and disordered eating in adolescents: Longitudinal findings from project EAT. *Archives of Pediatrics and Adolescent Medicine* 162:17–22.

Myth #2: Your Body Shape Doesn't Matter

Canoy, D., et al. 2005. Cigarette smoking and fat distribution in 21,828 British men and women: A population-based study. *Obesity Research* 13:1466–1475.

Epel, E. S., et al. 2000. Stress and body shape: Stress-induced cortisol secretion is consistently greater among women with central fat. *Psychosomatic Medicine* 62:623–632.

Klein, S., et al. 2004. Absence of an effect of liposuction on insulin action and risk factors for coronary heart disease. *New England Journal of Medicine* 350:2549–2557.

Kohrt, W. M., et al. 1992. Exercise training improves fat distribution patterns in 60- to 70-year-old men and women. *Journal of Gerontology* 47:M99–105.

Lakka, H. M., et al. 2002. Abdominal obesity is associated with increased risk of acute coronary events in men. *European Heart Journal* 23:706–713.

Paniagua, J. A., et al. 2007. Monounsaturated fat-rich diet prevents central body fat distribution and decreases postprandial adiponectin expression induced by a carbohydrate-rich diet in insulin-resistant subjects. *Diabetes Care* 30: 1717–1723.

Rimm, A. A., et al. 1988. A weight shape index for assessing risk of disease in 44,820 women. *Journal of Clinical Epidemiology* 41:459–465.

Roberts, S. B., and J. Mayer. 2000. Holiday weight gain: Fact or fiction? *Nutrition Reviews* 58:378–379.

Schmitz, K. H., et al. 2007. Strength training and adiposity in premenopausal women: Strong, healthy, and empowered study. *American Journal of Clinical Nutrition* 86:566–572.

Whitmer, R. A. 2007. The epidemiology of adiposity and dementia. *Current Alzheimer Research* 4:117–122.

Myth #3: Calories Don't Count

Kennedy, E. T., et al. 2001. Popular diets: Correlation to health, nutrition, and obesity. *Journal of the American Dietetic Association* 101:411–420.

Sacks, F. M., et al. 2009. Comparison of weight-loss diets with different compositions of fat, protein, and carbohydrates. *New England Journal of Medicine* 360:859–873.

Leibel, R. L., et al. 1992. Energy intake required to maintain body weight is not affected by wide variation in diet composition. *American Journal of Clinical Nutrition* 55:350–355.

Rolls, B. J., et al. 2004. Salad and satiety: Energy density and portion size of a first-course salad affect energy intake at lunch. *Journal of the American Dietetic Association* 104:1570–1576.

Yunsheng, M., et al. 2007. A dietary quality comparison of popular weight-loss plans. *Journal of the American Dietetic Association* 107:1786–1791.

Myth #4: Carbs Are Bad for You

Giovannucci, E., et al. 2006. A prospective study of calcium intake and incident and fatal prostate cancer. *Cancer Epidemiology, Biomarkers & Prevention* 15:203–210.

Marsh, A. G., et al. 1988. Vegetarian lifestyle and bone mineral density. *American Journal of Clinical Nutrition* 48(3 Suppl.):837–841.

Myth #5: Carbs Are Good for You

Mattes, R. D. 2002. Ready-to-eat cereal used as a meal replacement promotes weight loss in humans. *Journal of the American College of Nutrition* 21:570–577.

Presutti, R. J., et al. 2007. Celiac disease. *American Family Physician* 76:1795–1802.

PR Newswire Association, 2005. Raisins at Halloween treat kids to healthy teeth. News release, California Raisin Board, October 20.

Stanhope, K. L., and P. J. Havel. 2008. Fructose consumption: Potential mechanisms for its effects to increase visceral adiposity and induce dyslipidemia and insulin resistance. *Current Opinion in Lipidology* 19:16–24.

Waller, S. M., et al. 2004. Evening ready-to-eat cereal consumption contributes to weight management. *Journal of the American College of Nutrition* 23:316–321.

Myth #6: Diet Drugs Are a Magic Bullet

Anderson, J. W. 2008. Orlistat for the management of overweight individuals and obesity: A review of potential for the 60-mg, over-the-counter dosage. *Expert Opinion on Pharmacotherapy* 8: 1733–1742.

Bray, G. A. 2008. Are non-prescription medications needed for weight control? *Obesity* 16:509–514.

Ioannides-Demos, L. L., et al. 2006. Safety of drug therapies used for weight loss and treatment of obesity. *Drug Safety* 29:277–302.

Neff, L. M., and L. J. Aronne. 2007. Pharmacotherapy for obesity. *Current Atherosclerosis Reports* 9:454–462.

Rosenstock, J., et al. 2008. The SERENADE Trial: Effects of monotherapy with rimonabant, the first selective CB1 receptor antagonist, on glycemic control, body weight and lipid profile in drug-naive type 2 diabetes. *Diabetes Care* 31:2169–2176.

Rubio, M. A., et al. 2007. Drugs in the treatment of obesity: Sibutramine, orlistat and rimonabant. *Public Health Nutrition* 10(10A): 1200–1205.

Schwarz, S. M., et al. 2008. Compliance, behavior change, and weight loss with orlistat in an over-the-counter setting. *Obesity* 16:623–629.

Wacker, D. A., and K. J. Miller. 2008. Agonists of the serotonin 5-HT2C receptor: Preclinical and clinical progression in multiple diseases. *Current Opinion in Drug Discovery and Development* 11:438–445.

Wall, J. V., et al. 2008. Egg breakfast enhances weight loss. *International Journal of Obesity* 32:1545–1551.

Myth #7: Dieting Is All You Need to Lose Weight

Bravata, D. M., et al. 2007. Using pedometers to increase physical activity and improve health: A systematic review. *Journal of the American Medical Association* 298:2296–2304.

Economos, C. D., et al. 2007. A community intervention reduces BMI z-score in children: Shape Up Somerville first year results. *Obesity* 15:1325–1336.

Shaw, K., et al. 2006. Exercise for overweight or obesity. *Cochrane Database of Systematic Reviews* October 18:CD003817.

Myth #8: Supplements Will Make You Thin and Healthy

Bejakovic, G., et al. 2007. Mortality in randomized trials of antioxidant supplements for primary and secondary prevention: Systematic review and meta-analysis. *Journal of the American Medical Association* 297:842–857.

Bowerman, S. 2006. Meal replacements for weight management: Carefully chosen bars and shakes can be valuable. *Advance for Nurse Practitioners* 14:37–39, 65.

Bui, L. T., et al. 2006. Blood pressure and heart rate effects following a single dose of bitter orange. *Annals of Pharmacotherapy* 40:53–57.

Douglas, R. M., et al. 2007. Vitamin C for preventing and treating the common cold. *Cochrane Database of Systematic Reviews* 18: CD000980.

Huang, H. I., et al. 2006. The efficacy and safety of multivitamin and mineral supplement use to prevent cancer and chronic disease in adults: A systematic review for a National Institutes of Health state-of-the-science conference. *Annals of Internal Medicine* 145:372–385.

Izzo, A. A., and Ernst, E. 2001. Interactions between herbal medicines and prescribed drugs: A systematic review. *Drugs* 61:2163–2175.

Kleijnen, J., et al. 1991. Clinical trials of homoeopathy. *British Medical Journal* 302:316–323.

Lawson, K. A., et al. 2007. Multivitamin use and risk of prostate cancer in the National Institutes of Health–AARP Diet and Health Study. *Journal of the National Cancer Institute* 99:754–764.

Lonn, E., et al. 2005. Effects of long-term vitamin E supplementation on cardiovascular events and cancer: A randomized controlled trial. *Journal of the American Medical Association* 293: 1338–1347.

Omenn, G. S. 1996. Risk factors for lung cancer and for intervention effects in CARET, the Beta-Carotene and Retinol Efficacy Trial. *Journal of the National Cancer Institute* 88:1550–1559.

Rosendaal, R. M., et al. 2008. Effect of glucosamine sulfate on hip osteoarthritis: A randomized trial. *Annals of Internal Medicine* 148:268–277.

Rothman, K. J., et al. 1995. Teratogenicity of high vitamin A intake. *New England Journal of Medicine* 333:1369–1373.

Saper, R. B., et al. 2004. Common dietary supplements for weight loss. *American Family Physician* 70:1731–1738.

Stranges, S., et al. 2007. Effects of long-term selenium supplementation on the incidence of type 2 diabetes: A randomized trial. *Annals of Internal Medicine* 147:217–223.

Myth #9: Low-Fat Diets Are a Waste of Time

Barberger-Gateaux, P., et al. 2007. Dietary patterns and risk of dementia: The three-city cohort study. *Neurology* 69:1921–1930.

Beresford, S. A., et al. 2006. Low-fat dietary pattern and risk of colorectal cancer: The Women's Health Initiative Randomized Controlled Dietary Modification Trial. *Journal of the American Medical Association* 295:643–654.

Fung, T. T., et al. 2008. Adherence to a DASH-style diet and risk of coronary heart disease and stroke in women. *Archives of Internal Medicine* 168:713–720.

Golay, A., et al. 2000. Similar weight loss with low-energy food combining or balanced diets. *International Journal of Obesity and Related Metabolic Disorders* 24:492–496.

Howard, B. V., et al. 2006. Low-fat dietary pattern and risk of cardiovascular disease: The Women's Health Initiative Randomized Controlled Dietary Modification Trial. *Journal of the American Medical Association* 295:655–666.

Kolata, G. 1998. Scientist at work: Dean Ornish; a promoter of programs to foster heart health. *New York Times*, December 29.

Ornish, D. 1998. Avoiding revascularization with lifestyle changes: The Multicenter Lifestyle Demonstration Project. *American Journal of Cardiology* 82:72T–76T.

Petot, G. J., and R. P. Friedland. 2004. Lipids, diet and Alzheimer disease: An extended summary. *Journal of the Neurological Sciences* 226:31–33.

Prentice, R. L., et al. 2006. Low-fat dietary pattern and risk of invasive breast cancer: The Women's Health Initiative Randomized Controlled Dietary Modification Trial. *Journal of the American Medical Association* 295:629–642.

Shai, I., et al. 2008. Weight loss with a low-carbohydrate, Mediterranean, or low-fat diet. *New England Journal of Medicine* 359: 229–241.

Thibaut, A. C., et al. 2007. Dietary fat and postmenopausal invasive breast cancer in the National Institutes of Health–AARP Diet and Health Study cohort. *Journal of the National Cancer Institute* 99:451–462.

Trichopoulou, A., et al. 1995. Consumption of olive oil and specific food groups in relation to breast cancer risk in Greece. *Journal of the National Cancer Institute* 87:110–116.

Myth #10: You Can't Keep Weight Off

Andrade, A. M., et al. 2008. Eating slowly led to decreases in energy intake within meals in healthy women. *Journal of the American Dietetic Association* 108:1186–1191.

Butryn, M. L., et al. 2007. Consistent self-monitoring of weight: A key component of successful weight loss maintenance. *Obesity* 15:3091–3096.

Catenacci, V. A., et al. 2008. Physical activity patterns in the National Weight Control Registry. *Obesity* 16:153–161.

Daeninick, E., and M. Miller. 2006. What can the National Weight Control Registry teach us? *Current Diabetes Reports* 6:401–404.

Fritsch, J. 1999. 95% regain lost weight. Or do they? *New York Times*, May 25.

Svetkey, L. P., et al. 2008. Comparison of strategies for sustaining weight loss: The Weight Loss Maintenance Randomized Controlled Trial. *Journal of the American Medical Association* 299: 1139–1148.

Wyatt, H. R., et al. 2002. Long-term weight loss and breakfast in subjects in the National Weight Control Registry. *Obesity Research* 10:78–82.

Index

About the Author

Dr. Nancy L. Snyderman joined NBC News as the chief medical editor in September 2006. Her reports appear on *Today,* NBC *Nightly News* with Brian Williams, *Dateline* NBC, MSNBC, and MSNBC.com.

Dr. Snyderman has reported on wide-ranging medical topics affecting both men and women and has traveled extensively, reporting from many of the world's most troubled areas. She is on staff in the Department of the Otolaryngology–Head and Neck Surgery at the University of Pennsylvania.

Prior to joining NBC News, Dr. Snyderman served as vice president of consumer education for the health care corporation Johnson & Johnson. There she led the independent educational initiative Understanding Health, focusing on educating and informing the public about health and medicine. Before that, she served as the medical correspondent for ABC News for seventeen years and was a contributor to *20/20, Primetime,* and *Good Morning America.* Prior to leaving ABC she was a frequent substitute co-host on *Good Morning America.* Committed to patient education,

Dr. Snyderman cofounded Lluminari, Inc., a Wilmington-based company that provides expert content to Fortune 500 companies on health topics.

Dr. Snyderman attended medical school at the University of Nebraska and continued with residencies in pediatrics and ear, nose, and throat surgery at the University of Pittsburgh. She joined the surgical staff at the University of Arkansas in 1983 and began her broadcasting career shortly afterward at KATV, the ABC affiliate in Little Rock, Arkansas.

Snyderman's medical work has been widely published in peer review journals, and she is the recipient of numerous research grants from the American Cancer Society, the Kellogg Foundation, and the American Academy of Otolaryngology–Head and Neck Surgery. She has received numerous awards for her broadcasting. She is the author of *Dr. Nancy Snyderman's Guide to Good Health for Women over Forty*, *Necessary Journeys*, *Girl in the Mirror: Mothers and Daughters in the Years of Adolescence*, and *Medical Myths That Can Kill You: And the 101 Truths That Will Save, Extend, and Improve Your Life*.

Snyderman lives in Princeton, New Jersey, with her husband, Doug, and is the mother of three children, Kate, Rachel, and Charlie.

Also by Nancy L. Snyderman, M.D.

MEDICAL NEWS THIS DOCTOR

WANTS YOU TO KNOW

MYTH: Vaccinations are just for kids.
FACT: More than 500,000 adults get
shingles each year. It can be prevented
by getting a shingles vaccine in
adulthood.

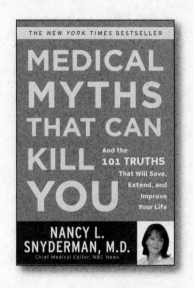

MYTH: Vitamin C prevents colds.
FACT: It can actually be harmful when
taken in large doses over long periods of
time.

MYTH: If I'm not overweight, I'm not at
risk of heart attack.
FACT: Thin people die of heart attacks
every day. The real culprits are smoking,
cholesterol, and triglycerides.

Stop diagnosing yourself with false information and half-
truths found on sketchy websites. In *Medical Myths That Can
Kill You*, Dr. Nancy L. Snyderman, chief medical editor for
NBC News, provides clear, practical, scientifically proven advice that can lead you to a healthier, happier life.

Medical Myths That Can Kill You:
And the 101 Truths That Will Save,
Extend, and Improve Your Life

$14.95 paperback (Canada: $17.50)
ISBN 978-0-307-40614-9

Available from Three Rivers Press wherever books are sold